stay fit and
fantastic
over 50

stay fit and fantastic over 50

jack hay

foulsham

LONDON • NEW YORK • TORONTO • SYDNEY

foulsham

The Publishing House, Bennetts Close, Cippenham, Slough,
Berkshire, SL1 5AP, England

ISBN 0-572-02887-3

Copyright © 2003 Jack Hay

The moral right of the author has been asserted.

Cover photograph © Powerstock

Neither the editors of W. Foulsham & Co. Ltd nor the
author nor the publisher takes responsibility for any
possible consequences from any treatment, procedure, test,
exercise, action or application of medication or preparation
by any person reading or following the information in this
book. The publication of this book does not constitute the
practice of medicine, and this book does not attempt to
replace any diet or instructions from your doctor. The
author and publisher advise the reader to check with a
doctor before administering any medication or undertaking
any course of treatment or exercise.

Printed in Great Britain by Creative Print and Design (Wales), Ebbw Vale

Contents

Acknowledgements

I would like to thank my wife, Sue, for the unstinting help and encouragement she provided with the researching and writing of this book, and especially for being a wonderful sounding-board for the original concept.

I would also like to thank all those health writers, doctors, nutritionists and fitness experts who were so supportive during the time when we were publishing *Good Health* magazine, and who now help with SlimSeekers, our weight-loss consultancy. Their expertise helped provide much of the background knowledge and information to be found in these pages.

Finally, a very special thanks to Wendy Hobson, Foulsham's editorial director, who guided the book through the publishing maze, and to editor Gill Holloway, who helped put my text into order, and offered yet another woman's perspective!

Introduction

The fact that you are reading this book suggests your age may be near that special milestone of 50 years. Alternatively, perhaps, you are simply curious about anything that could help you to live a longer and happier life. Well, you have undoubtedly made the right decision. Within the pages of this book, you will find the means to slow down your ageing process – and to maintain a healthier lifestyle that will give you more vitality than you have enjoyed for years.

There is no secret recipe for longevity. But many areas of our lifestyle influence how long we live, and in this book we will identify and define them, then show you how to take action in those areas in a coherent way with the aim of adding at least another ten years to your life. Not a bad investment for the price of this book.

If you are aged 50 or over, you have already seen quite a few changes during your lifetime. You may have been a passenger on the first jet airliner, seen the first film in Cinemascope, used the first non-stick saucepan, or driven one of the very first Minis. You will have seen the arrival of the heart pace-maker, the birth control pill, the microwave oven, satellite TV and the first portable music cassette players. You will have watched the first man step on to the moon. The last 20 years have brought a flood of new inventions – pocket calculators and home computers, video recorders, CDs, DNA fingerprinting, e-mail and internet access, mobile telephones and, the most important of all, the TV remote control! All of these were unknown to our parents when they were young, and yet our children take them all for granted.

You can slow down your ageing process and enjoy a healthier, more vital lifestyle.

The largest section of the population is now aged over 50 and the numbers are growing fast. In the year 2000 there were around 600 million people in the world aged 60 or over. There will be 1.2 **billion** by 2025.

The question is: how do we actively encourage nature to make us live longer? And more importantly, how do we make the most of these extra years? There is no point in being given a present if you can't open and enjoy it. And that's what this book sets out to do: to help you to achieve increased longevity – and to make the most of it!

CHAPTER I

Ageing

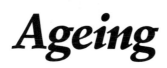

The search for long life has been evident throughout history, with folklore and legends telling stories of quests for the elixir of life or the fountains of youth. Magic water, rare fruits or plants and even precious stones have all played leading roles in legends over the centuries. As recently as in the last century a popular theory evolved that the bacteria in live yoghurt could extend our lives – and while it is certainly true that yoghurt has many healthy attributes, longevity has yet to be proven to be one of them.

In fact, of the many products that claim anti-ageing properties, none has been scientifically proven to work. Take, for example, the many very expensive creams on the market that claim to reverse the ageing of the skin. Although their claims cannot be proven, people still buy them, more in hope than any belief. It is too easy to convince ourselves that something will work for us, and so be exploited by clever marketing messages.

The sooner you start to address the factors that affect ageing, the sooner you'll see results.

Eastern concepts of ageing are more philosophical and embrace holistic health. Early theories evolving the balancing of *yin* and *yang* energies form the basis of Chinese medicine. Some ancient Indian philosophies recommend exercise, a balanced diet and the preservation of a calm and relaxed attitude.

So what does influence ageing? We in the Western world now know that attitude, genes, diet and nutrition, exercise, mental activity and stress are just some of the many factors that **do** affect your longevity and continuing good health. That means there are plenty of different ways in which you can add more years to your life. More importantly, you can put more life into your years, by adopting simple measures or philosophies to help reduce the effects of ageing. For example, people who are generally optimistic and positive about their advancing age are 19 per cent **less** likely to die prematurely than people who fear the idea of getting old – this is a fact established by the Age Research Centre in the USA.

Achieving optimum life expectancy

The optimum physical life span of a human is believed to be around 120 years, although people who reach this age are indeed a rarity. Before 1900, 75 per cent of people died before they reached the age of 65; and in the 1850s less than 5 per cent of the population in the UK was aged 65 or over. Today, on average, a man will reach 75 years or more and a woman 85 years.

We start 'ageing' the moment we are born. Babies have a fast growth spurt up until the age of around two and a second period of fast growth starts at puberty and progresses until around 20 years of age, with all of our body growth complete by around the age of 25. Up to the age of 30 there is generally a progressive increase in the power of both mind and body. It is after this age that a gradual decline in physical and mental vigour may begin, and such decline is normally related closely to the individual's lifestyle. Most people do not actually experience any decline until they are in their forties or fifties or, for a lucky few, their sixties. Even then, while physical capacity may decrease, mental capacity can continue to increase. In fact, some people's mental capacity can reach a peak in their fifties or sixties before starting to tail off.

It is thought that the speed at which we age relates to the deterioration of our body's cells over a lifetime of wear and tear, or it may be simply that nature has a cut-off point for each of us. But, of course, we do not all live in the same way or in a similar environment, and we all have to face various demands at different stages of our lives. For example, the stresses that we may encounter can and do affect our physical health and may therefore have a negative impact on the rate at which we age. Health problems such as heart disease have increased in the Western world over the last century, largely as a result of poor diet and lifestyle.

We already have a preconceived idea of what age represents and we may be ageist in our attitude to people without even realising. For example, we will readily identify friends or relatives whom we think of as 'old'. This is usually based on a summarisation of the person's physical appearance: the style, colour and quantity of their hair, the type or style of clothes they wear, their general demeanour. Interestingly, it has little to do with actual age.

Our chronological age affects us all equally, telling us the number of years we have been on this earth. But our biological age is shown by the physical and mental signs of ageing, and this will always vary from one individual to another. A mentally active 70-year-old may be far more mentally alert than someone a decade younger. Similarly, a 50-year-old who has kept physically fit will be able to run faster or further than a 30-year-old who is overweight, smokes and has never bothered to exercise. So while we can't do a thing about our chronological age – except perhaps lie about it! – we can influence whether or not we grow 'old' or just keep going longer.

Ageing influences

There are a number of issues that directly affect the speed at which we age. Understanding these issues is the first step towards slowing down our progress towards old age.

Genetic inheritance

The particular genes that directly influence our ageing process relate to the maintenance and repair of our body cells. Physical health, a tendency to put on weight, even our optimism (or lack of it) can all be part of our genetic inheritance. One thing we cannot do much about is the genes we inherit – and it is true to say that some people are dealt a better hand than others in this respect. For example, a rare genetic condition called Werner's syndrome is characterised by fast ageing.

What is under our control is what we do with our inherited characteristics. If we are naturally a bit lazy, we'll have to work that bit harder at the exercise part of the anti-ageing equation. We may not be as active as another person of the same age who is naturally restless and relishes being on the move, but then they may have a sweet tooth and so will have more trouble controlling their weight. We are all capable of making positive improvements to ourselves – if we want to.

Psychological attitudes

Perhaps the most important factor of all is our own attitude – our perception of how old we feel – and this is something we all have control over. Sadly, in our modern society we tend to dwell on the negative aspects of ageing, ignoring the fact that for many people, later life brings new challenges, freedom and new opportunities, all of which have a positive effect.

Your mental attitude to life is crucial and may actually prolong – or reduce – your life expectancy. How much you actually enjoy reaching middle age and beyond will depend on how old you **feel** – not how old you really are. So it is important to remember that ageism starts with your own thinking. If you start to think of yourself as older, you subconsciously come to accept the possible ageist attitude of others. You may start to see yourself as others want to see you, which may have little relation to the real you in terms of both physical and mental fitness. Before you know it, you will start to feel older than you actually are, and your demeanour, body language and even your clothes and style will adapt and change to reflect this old person that you imagine you have become, and you will end up old before your time.

Retirement in particular should be regarded as a turning point where you can experience new freedom, take up new interests, realise ambitions, and meet new people. Certainly, it is a time for positive changes. And if you expect new and interesting things to happen and actively search them out, they will be more likely to occur sooner than later. According to psychologists at Yale University in Connecticut, thinking positively about ageing can add, on average, a good seven years to your life. But worrying about getting older can take years off it.

The same experts at Yale concluded that taking a positive attitude was actually of more benefit than taking exercise, losing excess weight or quitting smoking, each of which can put between one and three years on your life. Personally, I would advocate doing all four, to try to add as many years as possible!

With your positive attitude you will know what is important to you. Your relationships, interests and responsibilities all combine to make your life fulfilling. Take pride in your achievements and don't think about past mistakes that cannot be undone. Look to the future with optimism and hope, and try to maximise and enjoy every new day that brings new challenges.

Mental activity

The way you use your brain will have a positive or negative effect on how quickly your mental processes slow down. Our brains require constant stimulation and they can be exercised and strengthened like any other muscle in our body. Older people often complain about increased forgetfulness and we've all had the experience of walking up the stairs or into a room only to wonder why we went there in the first place. Don't worry, there is something you can do about it. Making lists and organising your thoughts can help to improve the power of your mind – and your memory. Do crosswords, read books, talk to people – anything that exercises your brain may help to improve its function.

Physical exercise

There is little doubt that most medical experts believe the more our bodies are used, the more effective and efficient they remain. Resting the body just because we are getting older is not going to help its efficiency, although the amount of stimulation we give it must obviously be subject to our medical and physical limitations. Many people put down their lack of energy to the simple fact of getting older, but the most likely cause is that they are leading a more sedentary life as the years pass. Exercise is important at any age; we all need to put a little moderate exercise into our lives, not only for the sake of our health, but also for fun. The more exercise you can manage within your physical capabilities, the better you will feel, and the more you will want to exercise. Don't worry, this doesn't have to involve energetic gym workouts! Just taking a simple walk every morning will help to improve your energy levels. If you enjoy it and make it part of your routine, so much the better.

Diet and nutrition

The kind of food you eat will have a great influence on both your body and your mental well-being. You wouldn't expect a Mercedes to run at its best on paraffin, so why do so many of us expect a high-fat, junk food diet to keep us healthy? It simply doesn't make sense. A high-fat diet, combined with too little exercise, will make anyone overweight, an increasingly common problem in Western society and another ageing factor as it puts too much pressure on our bodies.

A balanced diet with plenty of fresh foods, fruit and vegetables is the best possible fuel for our bodies. A good diet will also provide us with antioxidants, which will protect cells by binding harmlessly with damaging free radicals (see page 15), making them impotent, so our diet should include as many as possible.

Stress

We all know that stress is bad for us. Stress can occur anywhere, but it is commonly found in the workplace and research now shows that the type of work we do may have a direct influence on our life expectancy. This has more to do with our mental state than any physical factors (it has nothing to do with occupations that are physically life-threatening, such as motor racing or mountain climbing). It is, quite simply, that those occupations with a higher life expectancy seem to be those that are personally fulfilling for the individual – and this can be at any level.

A little pressure never hurt anyone, but those of us who experience a great deal of stress at work are likely to suffer more stress-related illness and accelerated ageing. Recognising stress and controlling your workload will be an important factor towards the length of your life. Our ability to cope with stress is also important and this will vary between individuals. People who have little ability to cope with stress can suffer from anxiety and depression and will be physically ill more often. Those people who cope with whatever comes their way are often happier and physically healthier just because of their natural attitude.

If you have suffered from a lot of anxiety or pressure in either your domestic life or your work environment, now is the time to take control of your life and to focus on positive emotions. It is important to identify any stressful areas and to limit their effects. Learning to relax with a new hobby or sport or using relaxation techniques will help to readjust your mind and body into a different phase. It is important that you do not turn to eating, smoking or excessive drinking to try to relieve stress. The only effective cure is to remove the cause, and to be prepared to resolve any difficulties by airing emotions or problems in a non-confrontational way. If you find this to be particularly difficult, then you should seek the help of a trusted third party to intervene on your behalf.

Life changes

Changes in our life circumstances may also have an influence on how quickly we age. Amongst these are natural processes such as the menopause, which may bring sudden changes, both mental and physical. But changes in our lifestyle will also have an effect. One of the most important of these is retirement, which, paradoxically, can itself bring stress, suddenly increasing the ageing process. Some people, men in particular, find stopping work stressful. Once again, mental attitude is the important factor, and with the right attitude, retirement can be a real blessing. The important thing is to consider it as a beginning, not an ending.

Retirement doesn't have to be associated with being past your sell-by date. You don't need to consider yourself as having no further use. You may certainly have stopped the daily grind of commuting to work when there is no financial need to do so, but instead you can fill your life with things you want to do as opposed to what you have to do. This may include an interesting part-time job, voluntary work, or taking up an educational challenge. The social skills you have developed over the many years of a working environment will come into full force. Today, computer skills in the home will allow regular communication by e-mail and time to explore the world on the internet – just a fantasy a few years ago.

As mentioned earlier, sport can fulfil many ambitions while also helping to retain or improve fitness. Getting involved with a sports club through golf, tennis, bowls, bowling, or swimming, etc, can be time-consuming – and can fulfil both physical and social needs. Have a wander around a golf course midweek and see the number of 'veterans' enjoying themselves. No more crowded golf courses on a Saturday or Sunday for them.

The effects of environment

The cells of our bodies may be damaged by various environmental factors. One of these is oxidative damage, which results from attack by free radicals, the by-products of our body's requirements for oxygen. Our cells use oxygen to make energy, but sometimes this can be misdirected to other parts of the body, making us age more quickly. These fragments, or free radicals, are unstable and will bind together with the nearest molecule. Oxygen gives life, but it can also be negative – just think how it rusts metal, makes fat rancid and causes the browning of peeled fruits and vegetables. Oxygen put in the wrong place also causes us to age more quickly.

External factors can influence the body to produce more free radicals. Pollution, radiation and industrial chemicals in the atmosphere can all increase their production, as can smoking, drug abuse and heavy drinking. If we can avoid these elements, it will help slow down the ageing process. Nature provides our bodies with powerful antioxidant enzymes that guard our cells against attack by free radicals, but we can boost our natural defence mechanism by adopting a healthy and active lifestyle.

Your anti-ageing plan

Having established the factors that influence our ageing process, step two is to examine them in more detail. Read on and you will find the best ways of dealing with them to give you a longer, more active and healthier life.

18 holes anyone?

On a personal note, when I first took up golf in my late thirties I was amazed at the age of some of the women who played at the course on a Tuesday (ladies' day). One lady was 84 years old and had played every week for as long as anyone could remember. When she reached 87 she semi-retired – and only played nine holes rather than 18!

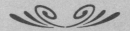

CHAPTER 2

Looking Good

The media today seems to be obsessed with people who are young and thin, and consequently most of us may be influenced into thinking that looking young and skinny is the only way forward. But in reality people over 50 years of age now outnumber the younger ones in the UK and elsewhere in the West. Moreover, just because you are over 50, you don't have to reach for a cardigan and carpet slippers. Remember, however, aiming to look and feel good is what it is about, **not** aiming to look 20.

At any time of life, our attitude to the way we look has a great effect on the way we actually look and increasing age tends to bring confidence in ourselves and our own style, leading to contentment in the way we physically look. We feel better about ourselves, so we look better.

Our financial situation may be better too. Our working environment may be less hectic and there may be less pressure as we head towards semi- or permanent retirement. All these things combined allow us more time, with a little extra money to spend to indulge ourselves in different ways of helping us to look good.

Naturally, most us would like to lose a little weight or perhaps a few wrinkles, but the important thing is to keep a perspective about our aims and ambitions. We can certainly influence our appearance by the clothes that we choose to wear, and we can all look and feel more healthy by adopting a good diet and fitness regime. These last two are so important, I shall deal with them separately later in the book.

Having confidence in your own style makes you feel better about yourself and helps you look better.

Posture

Sometimes the simplest things can make a major difference, and when we are talking about looking good, that is certainly true of our posture, as it has a major influence on both the way we feel and the way we appear to others.

Think about it. As we age, most of us start to appear smaller. Many people lose weight, bones and muscles become weaker and do actually shrink. So, simply by holding yourself tall and upright, you can immediately make yourself look younger – and you will actually **feel** different. Your clothes will hang better and you will appear slimmer. A big bonus is that good posture is good for your health in a variety of ways. Correct stance combined with regular exercise is believed to be the most effective way of increasing bone density and protecting the spine as you get older. If you are still working, you'll probably be one of the 50 per cent of office workers who complain of having some neck and lower back pain, usually through sitting at a desk or computer most of the working day. Constant slouching can give you a hunched back, rounded shoulders and allow your stomach to fall forward, making you appear bloated. Not so good at any age but definitely a minus when you are over 50 years old!

Correcting your posture

This is just a matter of getting into good habits – and in time, it will become automatic. Don't slump when you sit in a chair. Always sit well back so that both your back and thighs are supported. Sitting correctly will prevent your spine from becoming rounded. Try not to cross your legs, as this can inhibit circulation, and always hold your head upright to support it correctly – amazingly, it can weigh somewhere between 4.5 kg (10 lb) and 6.8 kg (15 lb), which is quite a lot to balance on top of your spine!

The Alexander Technique

A natural therapy used for establishing good posture is the Alexander Technique. Practitioners claim that learning to stand correctly and to maintain an upright poise can increase your height by up to 2.5 cm (1 in). The technique teaches you to undo all those bad habits developed over the years – such as arching your back and slouching, which causes your stomach to collapse or protrude out of the pelvic basin. Practitioners recommend at least a dozen supervised sessions to help achieve an overall good posture. They'll teach you how to lengthen your spine and loosen the limbs to regain a natural upright position. The instructor will look at how you naturally use your body and teach you how to protect it so you are not causing your muscles or your back any further damage. You may also work with your practitioner to deal with every day situations such as sitting in your car or working at a desk. (For more information, see Chapter 10, page 147.)

Fashion and style

Your clothes can age you – or they can take years off you. Slavishly following fashion is really for the young but there's no reason why you shouldn't develop your own modern, changing style. Your appearance should reflect what suits you best, giving you confidence and a self-awareness without making you look older than you are, or trying to look ridiculously young. As a good rule of thumb, if you are out shopping and think that the outfit you are considering would look good on a 20-year-old, it's a pretty reliable guide that it's not for you. Try to be objective when you try something on. Take a really long look at yourself in the mirror to see whether what you are trying on is flattering and makes you look and feel good. If you have a partner or friend that you can rely on to give you a truly unbiased opinion, take them along too – and listen to what they say!

Stand well to release tension

When standing, try not to slouch. At first, you may have to keep reminding yourself to stand up straight, but it will soon become easier, especially as your muscles strengthen.

Hold your shoulders back and lift your head high, as if someone is pulling the crown of your head up on a string.

You will notice a difference straight away as your spine straightens and your tummy is pulled in.

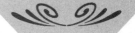

Depending on our body shape, each of us will find that certain styles make us look our best, emphasising our best features and disguising those we are not so happy about. There are plenty of TV programmes and books on finding the right styles and colours to flatter your individual shape and make you look your best, so use their advice to work out the ideal styles for you. Remember that what suited you when you were in your twenties is unlikely to suit you now. Go through your wardrobe and identify the items that you know flatter you – the ones that usually draw a compliment. If in doubt, get a brutally honest friend to help you. If there are outfits there that you never wear, it is probably because, subconsciously, you know they don't suit you. The contents of your own wardrobe will tell you what you should be buying and wearing.

Choosing clothes

As I said, when it comes to buying clothes, your choice will depend on your body shape and your individual style, but there are some general guidelines to follow. For women, if your figure has become fuller with age, it is more flattering to wear longer, tailored jackets rather than short, boxy styles. Skirts gathered at the waist will widen the waist and hips, so tailored skirts are more flattering; pencil skirts accentuate a slim figure and A-line skirts will disguise large hips. Look at the length of skirt that suits you best: avoid mini-skirts at all costs. No matter how good your legs are, very short skirts are not for the over 50s. Also avoid skirt hems that finish at the largest part of your calves – they will make your legs look thick. If you are a little overweight, don't go for tight, stretchy tops that show off every contour: looser-fitting ones that are subtly shaped into the waist will conceal the bulges more effectively. Heavy, stiff fabrics, particularly beaded or embroidered ones, are not a good choice if you are trying to hide a large bust. Go for a softer look: finer fabrics that drape well will flatter your curves without accentuating them. Finally, don't let yourself slink into the habit of wearing sensible flat shoes all the time – they may be very comfortable, but higher heels lengthen the body and show off good legs.

Men should take the same hard look at themselves. V-necked sweaters may be a staple of many an older man's wardrobe but they do emphasise drooping shoulders, so make sure you wear a shirt with a collar underneath or add some interest around the neck to distract the attention. Trousers should always fit well: too large around the waist and they emphasise thinness, too tight and they'll emphasise your belly – and, even worse, your bottom. The length must be right as well: if they are too short, they won't do you any favours at all. Double-breasted jackets and baggy trousers will add or emphasise width, whereas single-breasted jackets and slimmer trousers will add some height. Anything that is too tight or too brief looks plain awful, so if that's what's in your wardrobe, you must either lose weight or buy a larger size.

Colour is important too. A session with a colour therapist could make an unusual gift for a friend or partner's 50th birthday. Look at the effect of different colours on your skin tone. Those that compliment you will make you look vibrant, those that don't will 'drain' you. The effects of different colours will alter as your hair colour and skin tone change with age, so don't be afraid to change and adapt. Darker colours are slimming, but as we get older, some may be less forgiving. Large or fussy prints and patterns attract the eye, and so are best kept for your most attractive features and then only in moderation.

Style isn't about wearing designer labels, although you may well find that certain labels have a particular style that suits you. Style is also not necessarily about high fashion, although it is influenced by keeping up to date. Many people, especially men, do get caught up in a time-warp as far as their clothes and hair are concerned, without realising that sticking with an out-of-date style is actually ageing. If someone in their fifties is still wearing clothes similar to those they wore in their thirties, this is likely to be because it was probably the decade in which they felt the most confident in terms of both dress and style. They still see themselves as they did then – it will be others who will see the difference! Look at new styles, make changes, adopt those elements of fashion that show you are moving with the times.

Even what you wear underneath the clothes you can see will make you **feel** different. Modern underwear is usually far more comfortable, lighter and more attractive than its predecessors, and just the feel of silk or a lighter cloth against the skin can make all the difference to the way you feel inside. When it comes to buying a bra, it is worthwhile for women to have a proper fitting, especially as your shape may well have changed over the years. You don't have to go to a specialist shop – many high street stores offer the service free, and you may be surprised how much more comfortable you feel and how much better your clothes look when you are wearing the right undergarments.

You may think your entire appearance needs a complete make-over, or perhaps you just need a few gentle nudges in the right direction. Either way, go through your wardrobe, establish your style and take everything that is **seriously** unsuitable (too young, too short, too tight, too revealing) down to the charity shop. If you can afford it, splash out on a complete new wardrobe – but remember to take a long cold look at everything before you buy. If not, take time to apply the new principles gradually as you buy new clothes and discard the old ones that you know don't work any more. Remember you will always feel comfortable with what you are already used to, so it will take a conscious effort to make a change in style or colour.

Your hair

Changes to our hair are amongst the first visible signs of ageing. We all normally lose around about 100 hairs a day without anyone noticing (apart from when we clean the bath or shower tray). Temporary hair loss can also be caused by illness, certain drugs or nutritional deficiencies, particularly lack of vitamin A and the minerals zinc and iron, so any early hair problems can be worth a visit to your doctor. Hair lost in this way quickly re-grows, but permanent hair loss occurs when the follicles wear out and the hairs are not replaced. It is difficult to understand why some people lose their hair and others don't, but many experts believe there may be a connection between hair loss and hormonal changes in the body. Two out of three men can expect to be balding by 50 years of age and as many as a third of all women between 40 and 50 will suffer some degree of hair thinning or loss. Although hair loss is more pronounced in men, women will also experience a thinning of hair, which often occurs around the time of the menopause when oestrogen levels start to drop. In addition, recent research shows that environmental issues are causing both men and women to lose hair at an earlier age then ever before.

Choosing a hairstyle

Men with a full head of hair have plenty of choice but, as with clothes, sticking with the same style for years is not always the best option. You probably realise that you are unlikely to look great with the same cut as an 18-year-old, but keeping that style you had in the 1980s may be equally ageing.

If you are losing your hair, it is really best to accept your lot and adapt your hairstyle to suit. Today, this is not difficult, as many modern styles incorporate very short hair, and baldness is actually less noticeable with shorter hair. Don't try to grow your hair longer and comb it across to cover bald patches: it's much more obvious than you may think. Wigs are not much better – most can be spotted down the street. If you're embarrassed by your bald patch, ask your hairdresser's advice, look at magazines and styles and choose something simple, classic, smart and modern.

For most women over 50, long hair is a mistake, tending to draw your face down – which gravity is already doing for you. A shorter cut can take years off your face, and it will also emphasise your cheekbones. As we become older, hard lines are best avoided, especially in fringes, over the ears and around the nape of the neck, so keep the edges that frame your face softer. Whatever you choose, remember you are looking for a style that makes you feel good, is up to date but not trendy. Heavily styled and permed hair can add years, so try some of the new styling products and experiment with finger-drying your hair to achieve a soft and natural look. It is well worth having a chat with your hairdresser about updating to a more modern look that will suit you in terms of face shape and colour. It may also be worth going to a completely new stylist who will have no preconceptions of how you've worn your hair in the past.

Grey hair

Generally, grey hair can suit men, making them look more distinguished. For women, however – apart from a lucky few whose hair turns a perfect, delicate and utterly feminine white – greying hair is not very flattering and can seem much more of a problem. However, there are plenty of ways to disguise it, either by colouring it yourself, or having it done professionally. Highlights are a subtle way to hide grey hairs by blending in a lighter shade that complements your natural colour. If you have a complete colour change, remember that it is best to go slightly lighter than your original hair colour, otherwise it may look too severe.

Unwanted hair

In a cruel twist, as we start to lose hair on our heads, we start to develop hair in other places that we would much rather not have. With men, this tends to be in the nose and ears and you can keep a check on these when you shave in the morning. Any long hairs can easily be removed using special trimmers.

For women, facial hair may become an annoying problem. This is usually due to hormonal changes brought on by the menopause. There are several ways to deal with it yourself. Removing stray coarse hairs with tweezers is the simplest and cheapest but can very long-winded and quite painful. It is also only temporary and may even encourage the hair to grow back even more strongly. Depilatory creams will dissolve the hair just below the skin surface and should last for a couple of weeks. Always use a cream that is labelled as specially prepared for facial use (rather than legs, underarms or bikini line) and always test a small area on the skin first. Waxing is effective, and may be done at home or at a salon. The wax is applied warm, allowed to set, then pulled off with the hair – like pulling off a sticking plaster, and just as painful. It should inhibit re-growth and should last a few weeks.

If you prefer, you can have the hair removed permanently by a professional beauty therapist. Electrolysis is the most common method of permanent removal but requires more than one treatment. It uses a sterile electrical needle to kill each individual hair follicle with a tiny electrical charge. This more expensive method is long-lasting and quite effective, becoming more so after several treatments, but it can be painful and permanent removal will take some considerable time. A new faster method of removal by laser treatment is now relatively common. The hair follicles are treated with a small laser beam, killing follicles in small groups. This is highly effective but quite expensive, and treatment will still have to take place over a period of time.

Your skin

Young skin is supple, soft and attractive. It has a natural bloom that looks good with the minimum of attention. Older skin needs help to look good and the older you get, the more important skin care becomes. It is never too late to begin but obviously the earlier you start, the better the results. If you are still in your forties, there will certainly be some ageing effects showing on your skin, but how much depends on your genetic make-up, the amount of sun exposure you have had, your diet, lifestyle and skincare routine. By the time you are in your fifties, the skin of both men and women becomes drier, more sensitive and more susceptible to damage as the healthy cells are replaced at a slower rate. In women, the low levels of oestrogen after the menopause can slow down the rate of repair of skin cells dramatically, so taking care of your skin becomes even more important. However, there is no reason why at 50 years of age or over, your skin should not continue to be supple and soft – if you look after it.

To get the best skincare regime you can, it is probably wise to understand a little about the skin's structure, both inside and out.

Your skin is your largest organ. It weighs around 3.6 kg (8 lb) and can stretch up to 1.8 sq metres (20 sq ft)! Each square inch of it contains approximately 4.5 metres (15 ft) of blood vessels, about 100 oil glands and two kinds of sweat glands. Skin is totally waterproof – otherwise you would drown every time it rained. As well as helping to maintain body temperature, either by sweating or shivering, it protects the internal organs from infection and outside elements. It is strong enough to guard against injury, yet supple enough to allow our bodies to move freely. Amazingly, it is constantly renewing itself by shedding and replacing dead skin cells.

Our skin is made up of two main layers – the epidermis and the dermis. The epidermis makes up the top layer. These cells are continually replacing themselves with the old layer shedding as a new one pushes through to the surface. Teenaged skin renews itself every two to three weeks but when we are in our fifties it may take twice as long. The epidermis is where melanin is produced. This is the pigment that helps to protect lower layers of the skin from the harmful effects of sun rays.

Beneath the epidermis lies the dermis, a thick, cushioning layer that provides the overall strength and structure of the whole skin. The dermis is the layer that affects the way our skin looks and behaves and it is generally where the signs of ageing originate. The cells in the dermis do renew themselves but at a much slower rate than those in the epidermis, especially as we get older.

The main tissues that make up the dermis are collagen and elastin fibres. Elastin fibres are woven between strands of collagen to give strength and suppleness. However, the older we get, the harder it is for our bodies to replace these tissues, which ultimately causes the skin to lose moisture, become thinner and show the appearance of lines and wrinkles.

Taking care of your skin – on the outside

Whether you are a man or a woman, following a good skincare regime will make a great difference to the appearance of your skin. Men may recoil at the very suggestion, but there is no doubt that keeping your skin clean and not allowing it to become dry will help to hold back the ageing process. You don't have to go as far as buying special skin care products if you don't want to – washing with a mild soap and water and moisturising afterwards will do quite well. But if you do want to use skincare products, make sure that you select those that suit your skin type, bearing in mind that this may change as you become older. Many people find that their skin becomes much drier with age, and some women have problems with greasy patches and even acne during the menopause.

Women should take great care to remove all make-up before going to bed, and apply plenty of moisturiser both during the day and at night. You will have to experiment to find the products that suit you best, and do remember that the most effective products are not necessarily the most expensive – a huge amount of the cost of the latter is literally wrapped up in packaging.

Skincare products

The skincare product market is booming and companies are continually bringing out new ranges for both men and women, containing the latest ingredients that are claimed to combat signs of ageing. Truthfully, although creams can make the skin appear smoother, the chances of them actually penetrating the surface to the dermis and repairing any damage is unlikely. However, it is important to keep skin clean, moisturised and protected from the environment. Here are some of the main ingredients and what they do.

- **Alpha-hydroxy acids (AHAs)**   These act as a rapid exfoliant, loosening dead skin cells on the surface, and causing the skin to renew itself more rapidly. Although this can be effective, leaving the skin surface quite smooth for a short period, it can be harsh, especially on sensitive skin.

- **Antioxidants**   These are popular ingredients in many creams and include vitamin E. They work in a similar way to vitamins taken by mouth, but help to combat free radicals on the skin's surface caused by the sun and pollution.

- **Ceramides**   These are claimed to help retain the skin's moisture by creating a water-resistant barrier over the surface.

- **Collagen**   Applied in a cream, collagen is said to hold moisture in the skin by forming a resistant barrier, giving the skin a smoother, firmer appearance.

- **Elastin**   Extracted from cow fat, this makes a good moisturiser but is unlikely to penetrate lower levels of the skin.

- **Essential fatty acids**   When applied in a cream, these aim to hydrate the skin and so slow down the loss of moisture.
- **Liposomes**   These are claimed to give a longer-lasting moisturising effect, although the molecule size means that they are unlikely to penetrate the skin any further than the top layers.

Steaming
Simply steaming your face will cleanse it, unclog pores and get rid of unwanted blackheads, as well as helping to plump up the skin with moisture. You can give yourself a steam treatment quite simply at home: pour boiling water into a bowl and let it cool slightly, then cover your head with a towel and lean over the bowl, trapping the steam, for two to three minutes. Essential oils can be added to the water to encourage deep cleansing. Lavender and camomile are great for relaxing; frankincense and sandalwood are particularly good for sensitive skin. Afterwards pat your skin dry and apply a moisturiser.

Exfoliating
Exfoliating products, usually in the form of creams or gels, help to boost circulation, get rid of dead skin and speed up the rate at which cells are renewed. Put a small amount of the cream or gel in your palm and mix with a little water to make a paste. Gently massage over your face using a circular motion, then rinse off with clean, cool water, patting your skin dry. Always choose a product that suits your skin type and only use it once a week. Women may also like to buy exfoliating treatments to get rid of any rough areas of skin, such as on the thighs and tops of arms. These can be applied while bathing, using a sponge or loofah. (See also Cellulite, page 28.)

Taking care of your skin – on the inside
We spend literally hundreds of millions of pounds on beauty products every year in the quest for everlasting youth, but this is not the only way of improving the appearance of our skin. What we put inside our bodies is probably more important to the condition of our skin than the products we use on it. There are a number of nutrients that are vital for the repair and growth of skin, and ensuring they are part of your diet will give you a smooth and youthful complexion. Vitamins A, B, C and E are important as are the minerals copper, magnesium, manganese, selenium, sulphur and zinc (see Chapter 5 – Vitamins and Minerals). A diet that is rich in fresh fruit, vegetables and wholefoods will improve the appearance of your skin, as well as contributing to general well-being.

Nothing can replace the advantages of a nutritionally sound diet but if you lead a particularly hectic lifestyle and have poor eating habits, supplements can help to increase or maintain the level of essential vitamins in the body. A good multivitamin/mineral supplement will contain a balance of nutrients necessary for healthy skin and a number of companies are now actually producing specific supplements that are formulated especially for the skin. These can be found in most health food shops and chemists.

As well as what we eat, what we drink will have an influence on the condition of our skin. Most people who ladle moisturising creams and lotions on their skin don't realise that it is essential to drink plenty of water to keep the body and skin hydrated from the inside. Without it, the skin will dry out and show earlier signs of ageing. Although any kind of liquid will help (apart from alcoholic drinks, which can draw moisture out of the skin), by far the best thing you can drink is plain water, preferably filtered. Every one of us should aim to drink at least six to eight glasses of plain water a day. This may sound like a lot, but if you get into the habit of drinking at least one glass with every meal, then you're halfway there.

Pollution and severe weather can also damage your skin. A good moisturising skin cream will help to protect your skin from the effects of both of these and so it is a good idea to get into the habit of applying one every morning. Of course the greatest damage to the skin is caused by exposure to the sun, which is probably the primary cause of many of the lines and wrinkles you see in the mirror. But it's never too late to start protecting your skin. If you use a daily moisturising cream, look out for those that contain a sun filter. When it is particularly hot, use a high-protection sun cream – up to SPF (sun protection factor) 30 on your face, and at least SPF 12 for your arms and body – and wear a sun hat.

Changing bad habits
A well-balanced lifestyle will go a long way to keeping your skin in the peak of health – and it doesn't have to cost a fortune! There are lots of ways to improve the way you look just by getting rid of a few bad habits.

Smoking will accelerate the appearance of wrinkles, so if you do smoke regularly, try to cut down or give up completely, if you can.

Drinking too much alcohol will have the same effect, and we all know what we look like the morning after a heavy 'session'. Try to keep your alcohol intake to within recommended limits – 21 units per week for women and 28 for men (a unit of alcohol is equivalent to a small glass of wine, half a pint of beer or a single measure of spirits).

Avoid having too many late nights. There's nothing wrong with the occasional party or night out, but it is easy to get into the habit of dozing in front of the television simply because you can't be bothered to get up and go to bed where you can sleep properly. Your body needs sleep in order to repair and rejuvenate itself, leaving your skin looking fresh and glowing in the morning. The actual number of hours we each need varies considerably, but as a general rule you should probably aim to have at least seven hours a night.

Smile! This isn't as daft as it sounds. Some natural wrinkles are caused by facial expressions such as smiling and frowning – and you'll look much better with smile lines. You will also find that smiling will actually affect the way you feel – it's hard to feel grumpy with a grin on your face.

Take regular exercise. Believe it or not, exercise is good for your skin. Keeping active makes the whole body work more efficiently and increased circulation improves blood and oxygen supplies to the organs, including the skin, where it will help to enhance the overall texture of the skin and keep it healthy. Physical activity also helps to break down and disperse toxins in the body that can leave your skin looking dull. Finally, keeping in shape reduces tension and stress that can take a toll on the skin and general health in the long term, so it's well worth making the effort. (See also Chapter 7.)

Cellulite

Medical experts usually describe cellulite as fat and say that there is nothing you can do about it, as it is caused by the body's inability to deal with toxins under the skin, causing it to ripple. Beauticians and the manufacturers of beauty products disagree, of course!

Whether you are a man with a dimpled bum or a woman with orange-peel thighs, it's hard to know who to believe. But it certainly isn't worth paying possibly £50 or more for a pot of anti-cellulite cream or some other miracle cure unless you are sure it's going to work. And there are certainly cheaper ways to deal with it.

Some skin experts say that cellulite tends to run in families and the best way to avoid it is simply to eat healthily, exercise regularly, and maintain a normal body weight. They add that there is no scientific evidence that the various creams and moisturisers you see advertised have any effect: they may help to reduce water loss so that the skin looks plumper, but they don't really address the cellulite itself. Some clinics also recommend various kinds of massage. This may make you feel good but there is little evidence to suggest that it has any real effect.

So when it comes to cellulite, prevention is probably better than cure. Start with your diet: a low-fat diet with lots of fruit and vegetables is best if you are trying to avoid piling on fat. Try to avoid alcohol and caffeine, cut down on salt, sugar and junk food and take regular exercise. Keep off the cigarettes too. The same approach will help to reduce existing cellulite.

Secondly, regular skin brushing, which will help to improve the circulation and unblock the pores, should be carried out. All you need for this is a dry loofah or body brush – you can buy these in any high street chemist. Using long, slow strokes, brush the skin firmly in the direction of the heart. Start at your knees and brush your thighs in an upwards direction, working up to your buttocks. Brush upper arms from the elbows towards your shoulders.

Finally, lymphatic drainage massage can be helpful in dealing with cellulite. This should only be done by a trained practitioner. Special attention should be paid to the lymph glands, which are situated in the neck, armpit, backs of the knees and the groin. Essential oils can be used for the massage such as juniper, lavender, or rosemary. (See also Chapter 10.)

Your eyes

When we talk or listen to someone, we look at their eyes – it is our natural way of communicating. Our eyes convey a multitude of emotions and will be the first thing we notice about a person. Unfortunately, they are also one of the first parts of our bodies to show any signs of ageing and so care of your eyes is essential, both for the health of your sight and for your appearance.

Eye checks are essential for early detection of diseases such as glaucoma, which can ultimately lead to blindness. Most people should have a full eye examination at the opticians at least every two years, and as we get older, once a year, subject to your optician's recommendations. A small charge is made for this, but it is well worth the cost to know that any problems will be quickly diagnosed and dealt with.

Very few of us have perfect vision and a large number of people of all ages need to wear glasses or contact lenses to correct defects such as myopia (short-sightedness), astigmatism (distorted vision) and hyperopia (long-sightedness). If you find that you have to start wearing corrective glasses for the first time, there are many styles to choose from and your optician will advise on frames to suit the shape of your face, hair colour and complexion – and which ones to avoid. Do not put off wearing glasses because you think they will age you: modern frames can take years off rather than put years on. In any case, if you refuse to wear them and instead go round peering at everyone and everything, you really **will** look old.

Middle age itself brings a very common eye problem, known as presbyopia, which is caused by the loss of elasticity in our ageing eye muscles. This has the effect of making it very hard to focus on objects close to us. Most people first notice it in their forties or fifties, when they suddenly discover that they can't read a telephone directory or newspaper. Reading glasses are widely available from department stores and chemists in a range of different strengths. If you have no other problems with your eyes, just try out several pairs until you find the ones that suit your vision. However, if you are concerned about your vision or have tired or red eyes, you should see an optician. If you already wear glasses or contact lenses, it could be that you need to change the prescription, or you may need glasses for the first time. There may be a very simple solution, however. It may be the reading light at home that isn't bright enough – especially if you need reading glasses – or you have been sitting gazing at your computer screen too long. When you need to soothe those dry and tired eyes use lubricating eye drops. Avoid eye-whitening drops or any that contain adrenaline as this may be bad for your eyes if used over a period of time. A soothing eye mask is an excellent way of resting your eyes, or you could try laying raw cucumber slices on your closed eyelids.

Your teeth

Your teeth are one of the most important features of your face and without proper care will quickly start to show signs of age. Cracked, yellowing and decaying teeth are unsightly and gum disease causes bad breath. Not only does this make you look pretty unattractive, but it will also eventually lead to the loss of your teeth. Decades ago people accepted the fact that they would lose their teeth as they became older and dentures were fitted as a matter of course, but nowadays there are not many reasons why most of us shouldn't keep our teeth for life. You will have to give them some loving attention at home, and get some help from your dentist and hygienist, but it is well worth the effort both for your health and looks.

There isn't any alternative to a good brushing and flossing of the teeth, ideally twice a day (certainly for brushing). Dentists recommend using a brush with soft bristles rather than harsh ones, which can damage your gums. It is important to brush them for at least three minutes, using a circular motion, reaching into all the nooks and crannies, including where the teeth meet the gums, as this is where plaque develops. Use a good fluoride toothpaste and pay special attention to the tops and inside of the teeth, which are commonly missed, as people just concentrate on what they see in the mirror. The latest electrical circular brushes with interchangeable heads are very effective and some even have timers to ensure you brush for the correct length of time – usually two minutes.

Flossing involves sliding a length of waxed thread between each tooth to remove trapped food debris and break up plaque. If you haven't flossed for a long time you may need the help of a hygienist to start you off as some spaces between the teeth may be filled with plaque. If you find handling floss difficult, there are some gadgets on the market that hold the floss across two arms (like a catapult) so that you can use a handle rather than winding the floss around your fingers.

Whitening your teeth

A lifetime of eating, drinking and smoking can cause bad discoloration of our teeth, which can spoil the effect of a smile and the way we look. The best way to deal with this is a trip to a hygienist for advice on cleaning and the various procedures on offer. Special white resin bonding can be used to build up on to teeth enamel. In severe cases teeth can be cleaned and a thin layer of permanent veneer applied to the discoloured teeth, carefully blending in with other whiter teeth.

Most dental experts do not recommend the use of commercial tooth whiteners, as some of the pastes contain chemicals that can damage the enamel. Special products containing bleach can be used to remove mild stains but do not seal cracks in the enamel so stains can return.

Orthodontics

You may be unhappy about a crooked or broken tooth, an unsightly gap or a tooth that is severely discoloured. Both cosmetic dentistry and orthodontics have moved on greatly in recent years in terms of techniques and applications, and it will be worthwhile paying a visit to either if you have a nagging problem with the way you look. You will probably have to pay for the treatment as cosmetic dentistry is rarely available through the NHS, but the improvement in your appearance and self-confidence will be worth the cost.

Dentures

Most people's gums will naturally recede with age, so if you wear dentures you may need to have them readjusted for fit (and you don't want them clicking as you speak, do you?). Even if they feel comfortable, it is still worth having them checked by your dentist every few years.

Dentures should also be brushed regularly, with any remaining teeth you may have, to remove any build-up of plaque, paying special attention to the edges and the spaces between the teeth. It is also important to soak your dentures in cleaning solutions and carry out necessary everyday hygiene routines, to keep your mouth clean and fresh.

Cosmetic surgery

Not many people look in the mirror and feel completely happy with what they see. But the vast majority of us accept the physical flaws, considering them to be our genetic lot in life or simply the irreversible signs of getting older.

If you consider the typical person who would pay to have nips, tucks or implants, you'll probably imagine a rich American woman with an artificially bright smile, or a Hollywood star with large breasts. But the truth is that nowadays ordinary women and men (yes, men) are turning to cosmetic surgery to correct the parts of their bodies they simply don't want to live with any more. There's no typical profile of people who take the plunge but they all have a common purpose. They want to look and feel normal, perhaps by reducing an over-large nose, or lifting sagging breasts, or 'tucking' the rolls of fat round their tummy. They want to alter their physical appearance because it is constantly nagging at their confidence and self-esteem.

In the case of someone trying to hold back the years, the most popular are face-lifts, breast augmentation (or reduction), liposuction and Botox treatments for lines and wrinkles.

Reputable clinics

The easiest method of proceeding with cosmetic surgery is to go straight to one of the reputable private clinics that advertise to the public. The problem is knowing how to tell the difference between the reputable and not-so reputable that we sometimes read about. Your GP may be able to recommend one – you'd be surprised how often they are asked about this. If you approach a clinic direct, be certain that your consultation is with the operating surgeon or a qualified nurse counsellor, not a sales person who will later refer you to the surgeon. An advantage of seeing a nurse counsellor first is that it will give you the chance, in complete confidence, to discuss your innermost concerns with regards to your appearance. You can also find out the treatment options available to you and the pre- and post-operative requirements and expectations.

Even with the best surgeon in the world, there are risks attached to any kind of operation. Complications are rare in cosmetic surgery but post-operative infections, allergic reactions to drugs and dressings and even very serious problems such as deep vein thrombosis can and do occur.

To minimise any risks, for the weeks leading up to the operation you should be prepared to give up smoking – which increases the chances of post-operative chest infections – as well as to cut back on alcohol and to avoid aspirin, which impairs clotting. Some clinics may even ask you to reduce weight before an operation with the help of their dietician or nutritionist.

Be mentally prepared for any post-operative pain, swelling and bruising. Don't expect 'invisible mending' either – if skin is cut deeply it **will** scar: it's as simple as that. How well disguised or hidden the scars are depends on the skill of the surgeon. It's worthwhile approaching one or two of his previous patients to find out how they felt. This shouldn't be a problem with a reputable surgeon and the clinic should be happy to help you contact them.

Finally, don't expect miracles: correcting a physical imperfection won't turn you into a different person or solve all your problems overnight. But if you choose your practitioner carefully and have realistic expectations, cosmetic surgery could give you, like thousands of other delighted recipients, that little bit of extra confidence and self-esteem.

Below is a list of the most commonly-requested treatments. I have included some detail about the after-effects, which you won't find in the brochures.

Botox

This is a quick treatment to help get rid of lines and wrinkles on the upper part of the face, especially useful for frown lines and crows' feet. It only takes about half an hour to perform (hence the term 'lunch-hour' treatment), but it can be fairly expensive.

A tiny amount of purified botulism bacteria (Botox) is injected into a specific area near the line or wrinkle to be treated, where it binds on to the nerve, causing temporary paralysis of the corresponding muscle. Because it takes around three to six months for the nerve to start working again, the permanent lines caused by constant frowning gradually disappear. Over a period of time the lines will gradually reappear and the treatment can be carried out again.

There are very few known side-effects, but in a few cases where the Botox is injected near the eye, it migrates into the muscle that affects the eyelid, causing it to droop slightly. However, this usually resolves itself in a couple of weeks.

Other treatments that 'fill in' lines and wrinkles include the use of collagen, Restylane or Hylaform. Injections in specific areas restore elasticity and firmness to skin layers. This treatment usually costs less than botox treatment. Results and recovery time are immediate, with patients usually 'topping up' their treatment twice a year.

Breast enlargement

The surgeon makes a small incision (about 4 cm/1½ in) in the crease under the breast to create a pocket and then an implant or sac, filled with soft silicone, hydrogel or saline, is inserted. Some surgeons prefer to make the cut in the armpit or around the nipple area. The wound is then stitched, and a bandage or a special supporting bra is put on.

This procedure is performed under general anaesthetic, and usually involves an overnight stay in the clinic. The bandages are removed before you go home and a special bra will be fitted, which must be worn night and day for around two weeks, after which the stitches are removed. The breasts may be very sore for the first week and strenuous exercise should be avoided for about six weeks.

Implants can make it more difficult to get a clear result from a mammogram. There is a risk of post-operative infection and abnormal bleeding but these are rare complications. More common side-effects include hardening of the breasts and prominent veins, caused by the body forming a shell of protective tissue, called a capsule, around the implant. In this case the surgeon can manipulate the area to break up the tissue, although capsules can recur. Sometimes there can be a loss of sensation in the nipple area, but this usually returns in time. Despite early scares about the damaging effects of silicone implants, the medical profession nowadays is fairly united on the safety of this procedure.

Breast uplift
This does not make breasts bigger or smaller but shifts their position when they have become droopy, usually because of childbirth or weight loss. Before the operation, a new place for the nipple is marked out on the breasts. Under general anaesthetic, an area around the nipples is cut and skin from the lower part of the breasts is removed. The nipple is lifted to its new position and the skin brought together underneath. The wound is stitched and a padded dressing applied.

You can usually go home the following day. The breasts are likely to be sore afterwards, but the pain shouldn't be too severe. A properly fitted support bra will have to be worn night and day for several weeks and strenuous exercise and driving must to be avoided for a few weeks. There will be permanent scars, and there may be some change in the sensitivity of the nipples, but this usually goes away eventually. Some women may find that their breasts droop again at some time in the future.

Breast reduction
This may be carried out on both breasts, or only one if there is a marked difference in size. The nipple has to be moved with this surgery so the surgeon will mark out its new site before the operation. In very large breasts it may have to be removed completely and put back on. Under general anaesthetic, a cut is made around each nipple, then down and around the bottom of the breast. The lower part of the breast is removed and the nipple, usually still on a bed of tissue and attached to its blood supply, is moved to its new site before the wound is closed and dressed.

This is a major operation so you will have to stay in the hospital or clinic for two days afterwards, and will be unable to work for two to three weeks. The breasts may be very sore following the operation, but you will be advised on appropriate painkillers. You will have to wear a properly fitted support bra day and night for several weeks and strenuous exercise and driving are to be avoided for some weeks. Dressings must be kept clean and dry until they are removed, and after this time the scars, which are likely to be permanent, should be massaged with skin cream.

Liposuction
Liposuction is the traditional method of getting rid of areas of stubborn fat that diet and exercise won't shift, such as the face and neck, arms, legs or abdomen. It is usually carried out under general anaesthetic with a possible overnight stay in the clinic. One or possibly two small incisions are made in the area to be treated and a metal tube called a canula, about the size of a knitting needle, is inserted into the fat, which is then sucked out by a special pump or syringe. The small incisions usually only require one or two stitches each.

The area may be very sore and stiff for the first couple of days and you should try to rest as much as possible. You will usually be given an elasticated garment to wear over the affected area and this must be kept on for several weeks. After a week, the stitches will be removed and you can bath and shower again. Exercise can be resumed after around two weeks. There may be some numbness in the area, but this should disappear after a while. Results are somewhat variable – if too much fat is taken out or the skin tone isn't firm enough, there may be sagging or rippling of the skin and the patient may also end up looking lopsided, especially if that is their natural shape.

Liposculpture
Liposculpture is a more recent technique used for fat removal. Usually performed under local anaesthetic, subject to the size of the area being treated, the unwanted fat is carefully removed using a syringe and because the procedure is relatively simple, patients can normally return home the same day. Medicated saline is first infused through a small incision to saturate the fat, and the fluid and fat are then removed by suction. The small incisions usually only require one or two stitches. This technique can effectively reshape any part of the body, its sculpting effect helping to create a uniform line and smooth contour. It is not recommended for large areas of fat or people who are excessively overweight. Recovery time and conditions are similar to liposuction.

Tummy tuck

Also known as abdominoplasty, this is an operation to remove excess skin and fat from the stomach. Under general anaesthetic an incision is made along the bikini line and the excess skin and fat is trimmed away. The wound is stitched so the tummy looks as smooth as possible. You will normally have to stay in the hospital or clinic for two nights. The wound must be kept clean and dry and strenuous exercise must be avoided for at least six weeks. As it's one of the more painful of the cosmetic surgery procedures, you will be advised on appropriate painkillers.

Infection and build-up of blood or fluid can sometimes occur afterwards and the navel, which has had to be moved, can end up in the wrong position, which may require further surgery. There may be a loss of sensation along the scar, but feeling usually returns after a few months.

Face-lift

This procedure is popular with both men and women. Under general anaesthetic, the skin is cut from behind the hairline down to the front of the ear, then around the fold behind the ear and over to the back of the head. Excess fat in the neck, which may cause a double chin, can be removed and the neck muscles tightened so the jawline looks firmer. The skin is then stretched upwards and the excess cut off before stitching the wound.

Recovery normally requires one night in hospital. This isn't usually a very painful procedure, although the face may feel tight afterwards. You may be advised to wash your hair every day and an antibiotic ointment may be applied to the wound daily. The bruising should have gone down within two weeks and in two months the face should have returned to normal.

Occasionally the skin can get a very nasty scar called a flap necrosis. The precise cause is unknown but it seems to be more common in heavy smokers. There may be some permanent change in skin colour in the areas that were bruised. The hair can sometimes fall out around the incision, but it usually grows back within a few months.

CHAPTER 3

Feeling Good

If you think back to around 20 years ago do you remember waking up feeling refreshed, full of vitality, and ready to tackle the day with vigour? Does it seem, when you recall, that you packed more into a day than you do now in a week? Even then, you were having late nights and partying more than you should. So why the difference? Is it old age that is now creeping in and catching up? Is it pay-back time?

Developing a positive mental attitude really will give you lots more vitality.

The answer to those last two questions is simple. No. You simply have to make a concerted effort to get the vitality back into your life. A healthy diet and regular exercise are essential, and will go a long way towards gently persuading your body to cope with all the negatives life may try to throw at you. There's also an important mental factor in feeling good: you have to clear your mind of any energy-sapping emotional baggage that can lower your defences. It is all so easy, as we get older, to allow minor ailments, boredom, responsibilities and overwork affect our day-to-day lives.

The two aspects of feeling good – the physical and the mental – are almost inextricably intertwined. So, if you're in any doubt about your health, read Chapter 8, Good Health, and be happy with your physical well-being. It really doesn't make any sense to worry about possible illnesses that you don't have. And the other side of the coin is that if there is anything wrong with you, the earlier you discover a problem the more chance of dealing with it successfully. So logic states that it's a no-lose situation. And once you're sure your body is in good physical shape, you can concentrate more on getting your life into shape.

Managing your time

Many of us find that we are living our lives always half an hour behind schedule, both in business and domestic circumstances, which can easily become a habit over a period of time, and is both stressful and energy-draining, especially when we are in our fifties.

From a practical point of view, it is so much better to think ahead of the things you need to do, and to write a list of the items to be dealt with the next day. Subconsciously, this will help you to sleep well. The next day, go through your list and cross the items off as you deal with them, and any that are left over simply transfer to the following day's list. Remember, it is all too easy to expand any task to fill the time we have available, so be firm with yourself about the amount of time that you devote to any particular project, which will literally save you hours over a week. Enough to find some real 'pamper' time for yourself!

Using this method, shopping lists can also come into their own by helping you to decide what you intend to cook on a week-by-week basis, which will avoid those last-minute panic trips to the supermarket – or, worse, a quick take-away. And think of the money you'll save in food and petrol.

As we become older, especially with more time on our hands, we can easily become put-upon by influences from friends, family, business associates, committees and charities. Sometimes it seems easier to say 'yes' to everything because it is what you normally do, even when friends and family invite themselves to stay for the weekend. But, instead of automatically going along with other people's wishes all the time, wait a minute, and consider the situation. Do you really want to go through the motions and do something you would rather not do? It is important to be able to say 'no' and keep your commitments within your own requirements, even if you have to make some pretty lame excuses in your attempts to be diplomatic. You are not being selfish – they are. So there is no need to feel guilty.

Clearing the clutter

The older we are the more belongings we tend to have gathered around us. This may be the time to have a clear-out, which can be a springboard to all things new. For example, have you looked in your medicine cabinet recently? It's highly likely that most of the medicines are too old and out of date, and there are bottles at the back you don't even recognise. Throw them away and start again.

Check the wardrobe next. If you haven't worn anything for two years, you will probably never wear it again. Donate it to the local charity shop and create a load more space in your wardrobe for those new outfits (read through Chapter 2, Looking Good). If you haven't moved house for a few years or more, the garage and loft won't be a pretty sight. A day spent clearing either of these will bring you new satisfaction and put you back on the starting grid ready to get up and go.

Free your mind

Having a clear-out does more than put your house in order. It also helps to free your mind and emphasise the positive side of life that lies ahead of you. You will find that you enjoy life far more if you stop wasting energy on things that are unimportant. Plan ahead and make your time worthwhile, and retain quality time for yourself. Motivate yourself towards new challenges and always reward yourself for the goals you achieve.

Whatever you do, don't keep worrying about things you have no influence over, especially if they are in the past. Guilt can be a waste of time and an enemy of happiness. If you've done everything you can to rectify a bad situation, the best advice is to lock up your mistakes and throw away the key!

Your relationships with the people around you will, of course, have a profound effect on whether you feel good or not. If you are having relationship problems at a critical time in your life, don't suffer in silence – life really is too short. Chapter 11, Relationships and Sex, covers this in detail.

Fit to face life

Being physically fit will help you to deal with almost everything in your life more quickly and efficiently – that's why younger people tend, for the most part, to ride more easily over life's little problems. Fitness therefore becomes more important as we age, but it's a sad fact that it does require a little more effort to maintain our fitness on a day-to-day basis. In Chapter 7, Keeping Fit, I give full details on exercise and fitness options, but it is important at this stage to be singularly determined to complete some regular physical activity on a daily basis, or at least a minimum of three times a week. It may not come easily, but it is worth persevering; soon you will be physically and mentally stronger and feel a lot healthier, and it will help maintain your weight.

You don't have to go to a gym or embark on a fancy exercise regime. You could simply take a brisk walk in the park or along the seafront. Use this opportunity to breathe correctly and fill your lungs with clean fresh air. It will immediately make you feel brighter and it will also push out those harmful toxins (see Chapter 9, Your Immune System). Have a regular day out from home, and make the most of weekends. Go swimming, join a club and play tennis, golf or bowls, and if you have a partner, go together – you will encourage each other to keep going. Try meditation or the slow stretching exercises to be found in yoga, t'ai chi or Pilates. All of these can be done in the privacy of your own home, or, if you prefer, at classes. Great for both fitness and mental well-being.

Get into the habit of giving yourself a treat, especially at the end of a tiring day. Try an aromatherapy bath, using a relaxing essential oil such as lavender in the bath water. Or you can go for a luxurious bubble bath and obtain the benefit of the lavender essence by using special candle burners. Either way, it will be relaxing and you can even have a glass of sparkling wine to go with it.

We are what we eat

Our health and the way we feel is based around what we eat and drink. Our diet has an enormous influence on our health and well-being and that is why this book has whole chapters devoted to diet, vitamins and minerals, the immune system, and healthy eating. For now, bear in mind that to feel good you will have to eat a diet that is full of vitamins and minerals. Optimum energy foods include fortified breakfast cereals, fresh and dried fruits, yoghurt, green vegetables, lean meat, nuts, seeds, oats, pasta and pulses. Given the choice, always buy fresh organic produce to maximise the nutrient value.

Cod liver oil will help keep your joints supple and a multivitamin supplement with iron will help keep your energy levels up. Garlic and echinacea are also good herbal supplements to take to help boost your immune system, especially during the winter months. Also maintain those calcium levels, bearing in mind that skimmed milk offers just as much calcium as full cream milk, but with far less fat.

When shopping, try and get into the habit of reading (and analysing) food labels (see Chapter 4, A Healthy Diet). Processed foods contain sugar, salt and fat in various guises, along with colouring and taste enhancers, which may have a host of ill-effects, including giving you headaches, making you feel dull and adding pounds to your weight. The more you can do without them, the healthier your body will be.

Water is an important part of our diet and although we may drink it in various ways through tea, coffee and fruit-flavoured drinks, it is still important to drink around six glasses of water a day. Water assists the body's cooling system, aids digestion, removes toxins, and helps to keep our joints mobile and supple. As a bonus, it also improves the texture of our skin.

You are my sunshine ...

As the song says, sunshine makes us feel happy. This is not a myth – the warm rays of the sun actually have the power to make us feel good about ourselves, giving a psychological boost to our well-being. It provides significant benefits to both our physical health and our feel-good factor. It does this by stimulating the production in our brains of a chemical called serotonin, which is responsible for controlling our moods. So the more sunshine you are exposed to, the better you will feel. In addition, if you are enjoying yourself you are more likely to laugh, which in turn releases endorphins, the body's natural 'feel-good' chemicals that can help prevent many diseases. On the other hand, a lack of sunshine, especially in the winter, can cause a drop in our serotonin levels, triggering Seasonal Affective Disorder (SAD), a recognised form of depression. Research shows that you are less likely to die of heart attack in the summer, as higher levels of vitamin D (synthesised by sunlight) play a protective role for those people who suffer heart disease. One of the body's components in the skin (called squ-lene) is converted into vitamin D by sunshine, but without the sun it is converted into cholesterol, which may have something to do with the lowered incidence of heart attacks in the summer.

Vitamin D also helps your body to absorb calcium for strong teeth and bones. Scientists in the USA discovered that a daily dose of sunshine could prevent older women from fracturing their hips (a common symptom of osteoporosis). Several studies have shown that ovarian, breast and colon cancers are also slowed by exposure to sunlight. Vitamin D is stored in your body for the winter provided you get enough sunlight in the summer months – exposing arms and face at least half an hour every day from April to October.

We consume more salads and fruit in the warmer summer months, making it easier to reach our required five portions of fruit and vegetables every day for our fix of vitamins and minerals. Summer fruits such as strawberries, raspberries and blackcurrants are high in vitamin C with antioxidant properties to help against chronic diseases. They also benefit the immune system and, with their low calorie content, can help with weight loss.

Energy booster

For a quick, healthy energy fix, full of sugar and potassium, you can't beat the humble banana, especially useful after exercising.

As a slow-release carbohydrate, it will provide sustained energy that lasts, unlike sports drinks or chocolate bars that turn to fat if not used up through energy.

20 quick tips to feeling good

1 Have an annual medical check-up or healthscreen. A simple blood test can reveal so much about your health, and take any nagging worries away.

2 Eat a good diet with plenty of fortified breakfast cereals, fruit, yoghurt, green vegetables, lean meat, nuts and seeds, oats, pasta and pulses.

3 Devote 20 minutes a day to exercise. Take a brisk walk, use an exercise bike, swim, or follow a workout video. You will feel – and look – better.

4 Get an energy fix by breathing properly. Get maximum benefit in a clean air environment – in a park or countryside.

5 Drink plenty of water – at least six glasses a day, and more when you exercise.

6 Give your body a quick detox by eating only fruit and vegetables and drinking only water for 24 hours. Good for revitalising the system, especially after Christmas or a heavy party.

7 Clear your mind. Plan your day and don't waste time or energy on things that aren't important.

8 Retain quality time for yourself and give yourself occasional treats.

9 Motivate yourself to try new challenges and reward yourself for goals achieved.

10 Get into a regular pattern of sleeping at night. Avoid napping during the day, and avoid late-night stimulants such as coffee, alcohol or nicotine.

11 Get rid of clutter – clear out your wardrobe and the loft. You'll feel a whole lot better for it.

12 Be active. If you're going out with someone, don't just go out for a meal. Go for a stroll in the park or along the seafront or play a fun sport. Pretend you are on holiday for the day.

13 Try meditation and/or stretching exercises to relieve stress.

14 Start taking supplements every day – cod liver oil will help to keep your joints supple and a multivitamin pill with iron will help keep your energy levels up. Garlic and echinacea supplements are good for helping to boost the immune system.

15 Ensure your calcium levels are sufficient. Skimmed milk contains just as much calcium as normal milk, with far less fat.

16 Cut out those unhealthy snacks during the day. If you are partial to crisps and savoury snacks, try healthier alternatives such as pretzels or celery sticks dipped in low-fat natural yoghurt. Keep sliced fruit or vegetables in the fridge for hungry moments.

17 Don't presume that everything you eat is good for you. Read food labels carefully and cut down on take-away food and ready-made meals to avoid sugar, salt and fat, in a variety of disguises.

18 Don't have any worry or concerns about the past if you can't change the situation. Let the past go and move into the future, starting today.

19 Check your posture by looking in a mirror. Tell yourself you are the most graceful person on earth and watch yourself stand up. Now keep it that way!

20 Get out in the sunshine – it's good for you, so chase it if you can.

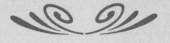

Controlled exposure to the sun's ultraviolet rays can relieve skin complaints such as acne, psoriasis and dermatitis. But it is better to walk around in daylight rather than sitting directly exposed to the sun for any length of time, because sunburn still remains a key factor in the cause of skin cancer.

We always want to get out and exercise more in the summer than the winter, which helps with the feel-good factor and our fitness. We run, swim and dance more in the summer or on holiday than in the winter months. The warm weather is also good news for those suffering with arthritis as it reduces pain and improves agility. Our blood vessels also enlarge, allowing for better blood circulation.

So plenty of reasons to celebrate the sunshine. A word of warning: however good it may make you feel in the short term, swimming and sunbathing without any form of protection are foolhardy. Whenever you're out in the sunshine, take care to use good sunblock products, loose clothing and wear a hat. You'll still gain all the benefits of the sunshine and warm air.

CHAPTER 4

A Healthy Diet

You are what you eat – so eat for health, balance and energy

If you are going to read and study any chapter in this book thoroughly, then this is the one. There is plenty of good practical advice throughout, but this is where it all starts. Because there is little doubt that what we put into our mouths influences our very existence, affecting our health, well-being and longevity – no more, no less. Unfortunately the word 'diet' has now become associated with slimming regimes and eating specific foods or, in many cases, the elimination of certain foods. But the term should and does relate to the food we actually eat on a regular basis, whatever that food may be. So we all eat according to a diet, but some people's diets will be a lot healthier than others. This chapter will explain what constitutes a healthy, balanced diet.

Making the most of all the nutrients that are available in our everyday food, especially as we get older, is extremely important. Even making a few subtle changes to your diet can quickly help to strengthen your resistance to many illnesses, from common colds to heart disease and some cancers (see also Chapter 9, Your Immune System). More recently researchers at Harvard Medical School discovered that a healthy diet that includes plenty of vitamin E may help in reducing the risk of Parkinson's disease. So it is worth knowing the various roles that different types of food play in looking after our body, and understanding how they work.

All foods can be divided into proteins, carbohydrates, fibre, fats and minerals, and we need to eat a balance of all of these to keep our bodies running efficiently. If you don't know your fibre from fat, or your carbs from coffee, then achieving this balance can be an uphill task, so read on.

Getting older

As we get older the balance of our everyday diet is even more important because our bodies become less forgiving. Our stomach will give us the hunger message when we need to eat, but some other messages such as lethargy, aches or pains and even stress go unheeded, and may be due to our bodies lacking nutrition. A poor diet can influence the health of our heart, and today's diets are often far too high in fat and too low in complex carbohydrates (see page 50). Nature cleverly designed our bodies to store fat when food is abundant (just like squirrels burying nuts) and today, when we do not experience any lean periods, our bodies still continue to try to retain the excesses of fatty foods that are readily available!

But why do we like foods that may be especially bad for us? Even when we may know that a particular food may not be particularly healthy, we still persist in listing it among our favourites – why is this? Obviously, nobody sets out deliberately to choose a diet or lifestyle that may be bad for them or to shorten their life. But our habits tend to evolve over a period of time, due to circumstances, family environment, youth, foolishness or poverty.

Our dietary preferences evolve from an early age and, subject to economy, most parents try to please their offspring with pleasant tastes and experiences. This may start with adding supplements to a dummy, like sweet water or a syrup to make it more desirable to suck. (And I can still fondly remember my grandmother giving me sugar sandwiches to keep me going until dinner time!)

This taste for sweet things stays with the majority of us for many years and then we discover a few unhealthy extras to add to our sweet tooth. These will be savoury treats (usually fast food), which will include hamburgers and chips, fried chicken, fish and chips, doner kebabs, Chinese and Indian take-aways, pizzas, etc. These form part of our social lifestyle at an early age, where we use the eating facilities to socialise with friends allowing us to be away from the home environment.

Even drinking alcohol and smoking tobacco are not usually taken up for their pleasant tastes, but because they represent all things adult, and there is no faster way than proving you are an adult by doing 'adult' things. Alcohol and tobacco are both addictive drugs, which will seem fairly sophisticated at the time, but can turn out to be very bad for us.

The threat of cancer and heart disease should be enough to put anyone off, but do we really believe it will ever happen to us? As we become older and wiser, this should now been the time for re-education and to throw out all things sweet, alcoholic, fatty or addictive. However, we have only just started, because our taste is fast evolving and we are still experiencing even more 'sophisticated' lifestyle tastes developed around convenience foods and eating out. Microwave meals from the local supermarket save a lot of time and taste good, and the variety offered is endless. Manufacturers will have tickled our taste buds with sodium (salt) and various flavours to make sure it has the texture, smell, appearance and taste to suit most of us. And those clever marketing people will have already persuaded us to buy it.

Convenience foods

Convenience foods are more expensive than a home-made meal made with fresh ingredients, but at the end of a working day who wants to work that hard? And after sitting all day at the office who wants to go out? A quiet evening in front of the television, a take-away or instant meal, with a glass of wine or lager, will do very nicely. The trouble is, although we may be working hard and paying to enjoy life's simple pleasures around food and drink, we are also fairly lazy when it comes physical effort. The car, taxi or train will speed us to our destinations. Television tends to govern our social life and getting up to pour a drink or load the dishwasher can be enough exercise for the evening!

Obesity with all its associated illnesses, heart disease and cancer all beckon. Are you getting the picture? At our age, we should be in total control of our lives – and want to remain healthy and extend our years for as long as possible.

Culture adjustments

People's eating habits are high on the agenda of nutritionists when compiling food and diet patterns over a population. Even within a single country there will be regional differences in what people eat, resulting from variations in climate. There will also be influences from other countries and cultures over a period of time, which will naturally be absorbed. In the UK and North America we have willingly adopted 'foreign' food into supermarkets, shops, restaurants and domestic kitchens over many years. It is not just the choice of food that changes via various cultures, but also the way it is cooked, seasoned and served. For example, chillies, olive oil, garlic and exotic spices are used in most domestic kitchens far more than 30 years ago.

Immigrant populations bring their own food culture with them, playing an important role in a country's food influences. Where once we would find a pub, a restaurant and a fish and chip shop on any UK high street, now there will be Chinese, Indian, Italian and French restaurants, along with take-away kebabs and burger bars. All these shops will now be the norm for current generations all over the UK and will influence our diet accordingly – and not necessarily for the better.

Income will also influence the types of food we purchase and variety of the diet we eat. In some societies it is actually a sign of wealth and status to be obese, but a more modern healthy eating philosophy is now significant in developing various trends and changes to cultures. As an example, in the last century brown bread was considered coarse and only eaten by the lower classes. Now wholemeal brown bread is known to be healthier than processed white bread and is actually more desirable, with its status increased.

Eating wisely

Although you think you may be eating healthily, it is a fact that the average person eats only half the amount of fruit recommended by the World Health Organisation but almost double the recommended intake of fat. Many people avoid breakfast or even lunch to stay in trim but then eat more snacks because they remain hungry throughout the day. Always bear in mind that we do not put on weight because we eat too much, but because we eat the wrong things.

Try counting the number of fruit and vegetable servings you have every day. You should be eating five servings but the chances are that you're not. However, when you read about the known benefits you may want to put this right – as from today. Carbohydrates, such as potatoes, bread, rice, cereals and pasta should make up nearly half of our daily diet, although the high-fat sauces that sometimes accompany them should be avoided. Meat is a good protein source but red meat is high in saturated fat and should not be eaten every day – chicken and fish are healthy alternatives.

You probably also have too many caffeinated drinks, such as coffee, tea and cola. Caffeine does give a mental boost, improving alertness and concentration, but only in the short term. On the downside, it can also cause the heart to beat faster and irregularly. Consequently, caffeine has been linked to an increased risk of high blood pressure, which can be more worrying as we become older.

Food diary

It is worthwhile keeping a personal food diary for seven days before you make any changes to your dietary habits. Just make a note of everything you eat and drink every day, without missing anything. Include every chocolate, every little chunk of cheese, every odd snack! Be clear about what you are eating and list each food separately. So if you have a sandwich, put down cheese, butter, white bread, etc. Describe the milk (full-fat, semi-skimmed or skimmed) and the type of butter or margarine (unsalted, low-fat, polyunsaturated, etc.) Don't forget to include spoonfuls of sugar in tea or coffee. Even when eating away from home, do not miss a thing (so that tube of sweets you ate on the bus has to go on the list too). Include everything – even if it is a glass of water, a squirt of tomato sauce or a smear of mustard.

If you can, describe how the food is cooked – boiling, baking, frying (sautéing), grilling (broiling), etc. and what it is cooked in, e.g. lard (shortening), butter, vegetable oil or olive oil.

Set out your diary in terms of time, place and whether you are with friends, family or on your own. If you can, include measures of food (knob, spoonful, ounce, large glass, etc.)

If you are really honest (and most of us are real cheats when it comes to dieting and food), your food diary will give you an excellent overview of your eating habits and will help you to analyse areas that you would like to change. You will be able to see at a glance whether you eat too much fat, or too few vegetables. Any bad snacking habits will be revealed and so will all those hidden calories that you hadn't taken into consideration – the spoonfuls of sugar, the dollops of cream and the extra slices of toast... It will also provide a clear pointer to any possible food intolerances or allergies that may be making you feel unwell.

Okay, so you've looked at your diary and decided you need to make a few changes to your eating habits. Don't just rush into this willy-nilly. To be really effective, any adjustment to an average diet will require some planning ahead, and you will have to know what you intend to eat and drink over the coming week, before doing the shopping.

It is also a very good idea to start informing yourself as to what ingredients are included in the food you buy. Reading a food label should not have to be highly skilled, but unfortunately the manufacturers seem determined to make it as difficult as possible. According to the British Heart Foundation, 20 per cent of people who read nutritional information on packaging find the content confusing or the print too small to read. Twice this number say they do not have enough time to interpret the information, and more than two-thirds say they need help understanding what it all means (see Food labelling, page 66).

A balanced diet

You will have noticed that when we talk about a healthy diet the word 'balance' keeps coming up. This is because it is important that we balance the intake of our food to achieve a number of goals. Our bodies need food from several different groups – proteins, carbohydrates, fats, fibre, vitamins and minerals, and plenty of water – all in different quantities. Eating healthily is not a matter of simply adding 'healthy' foods to our usual diet, or counting calories, avoiding additives or even taking nutritional supplements.

Choosing and eating a healthy diet involves knowing what mixtures of food to select on a regular basis (we all deserve favourite treats) and in specific quantities. It is important to understand why, so I have listed each of these groups of foods separately. We will cover the quantities later on page 53).

Proteins

Protein is produced from amino acids and is essential in the structure and function of all living things. Proteins provide the key building materials in all our body cells and are required for growth, repair and replacement. Eating meat, poultry, fish, milk, cheese and eggs, pulses, grains, seeds and nuts will provide our bodies with ample supplies of protein. Although meats are usually a major source of protein in the average diet, people who don't eat meat can get their supplies from cereals, pasta, legumes, nuts and seeds, eggs, dairy products and fish.

Carbohydrates

Carbohydrates supply the body's fuel or energy. Energy is measured in units called calories, and just one gram of carbohydrate contains 4 calories. They supply the energy for all your activities and keep things ticking over even when we rest. Carbohydrates are composed of carbon, hydrogen and oxygen and can be found in our diet in many forms, usually derived from plants. The healthier carbohydrates are called complex (or unprocessed) carbohydrates, such as wholewheat pasta, rice and wholemeal flour, and these contain both starch and fibre and supply the body with a slower, more steady flow of energy. It is best to avoid the carbohydrates found in refined foods such as sugar, biscuits (cookies), cakes, sweets (candies), etc., as these will be converted into fat for storage if not used in energy. See also page 65, Glycaemic index.

Fats

Contrary to what many people think, we all need some fat for our bodies to function. Fat is essential as an energy source and helps to insulate our bodies against heat loss and helps to cushion vital organs such as the liver and kidneys. Fat also acts as a carrier for vitamins and other nutrients. Stored fat can be used and converted into sugar to provide the body with additional energy when (and if) it is required. But there are different types of fat – saturated, monounsaturated and polyunsaturated – and some are good, and some are not! Saturated oils and fats definitely fall into the 'bad' category and should only be eaten in very small amounts. They are solid at room temperature, while unsaturated fats, which are much better for you, remain liquid. Almost all food contains some form of fat, with meat and dairy products being the highest in saturated fat. The fattiest parts are the streaks or layers of visible fat on meat and the skin of poultry. Processed foods such as crisps (chips), biscuits (cookies), cakes, pies and ready-made meals usually also contain high amounts of saturated fat. The fat content and the percentage of fat should be clearly marked on the food labels. Polyunsaturated and monounsaturated fats are the most healthy forms of fat; these can be found in fish, nuts and seeds.

A low-fat diet

I have said that your body needs fat. However, our Western diet contains far more than we need, so it is a good idea to cut down on fat as much as possible. Start by trimming all fat from your meat and removing the skin from poultry. Also use low-fat dairy products, and spread butter or margarine more thinly. Choose a low-fat spread if possible. When cooking, steam, grill (broil) or stir-fry rather than roasting or frying (sautéing) in fat. Use polyunsaturated fats such as sunflower oil for cooking, instead of butter or lard (shortening). Better still, use olive oil or rapeseed, which are high in monounsaturates. Oily sea fish such as mackerel, herring, tuna, sardines and salmon are all rich in (polyunsaturated) omega-3 fatty acids – which are highly beneficial as they can lower blood cholesterol levels. See also Chapter 6.

Fibre

Fibre is indigestible carbohydrate and is important for our health, as research shows that a high-fibre diet can prevent many of the diseases common in industrialised countries, including some cancers. Fibres act in the body in different ways, depending whether they are classed as soluble or insoluble.

Soluble, or viscous, fibre slows down the digestion of food and consequently the blood-sugar response, thus helping to prevent diabetes and high blood-sugar levels (hyperglycaemia). Also it is thought to break down fatty acids, thus reducing cholesterol in the blood, which will in turn help to prevent heart and arterial disease. Soluble fibre foods include oats, oat bran, peas, beans, root vegetables, such as potatoes, turnips, carrots, etc., and citrus fruits.

Insoluble fibre absorbs water, thus adding bulk to the material passing through the bowel, helping to stimulate the muscles of the lower digestive tract to move waste more quickly. It can help to prevent haemorrhoids and may also help to protect against cancer of the bowel. Insoluble fibre foods include wheat, rice, bran, pasta, wholegrain cereals, breads and nuts. Both types of fibre can be found in most vegetables and fruit.

Vitamins

Vitamins are vital organic compounds that we need for the growth, function, repair and maintenance of our bodies. They are classed in two groups – water-soluble and fat-soluble. Water-soluble vitamins include the B-complex group and vitamin C, and they need to be replenished daily as they cannot be stored by the body. Fat-soluble vitamins, which include A, D, E and K, can be stored in the body for longer periods. A balanced diet with plenty of fresh fruit, vegetables and cereals should provide all the vitamins your body needs. (See also Chapter 5, Vitamins and Minerals.)

Minerals

There are three groups of minerals – macrominerals, microminerals and trace elements. Macrominerals are required in larger amounts and include calcium, sodium and magnesium. Microminerals are needed in smaller amounts and include iron, manganese and zinc. Trace elements required in tiny amounts include iodine. A diet containing meat, fish, dairy products, nuts, cereals, vegetables and fruit will supply all the minerals you need. (See also Chapter 5.)

Water

Water is the elixir of life – our essential ingredient! Without it we would die in a matter of days. You should not underestimate the value of water and the important part that it will play in your healthy diet, well-being and longevity. It is very likely that you simply do not drink enough. An adult should be drinking at least six to eight glasses of water a day, depending on weight, age and level of activity. If you start taking regular exercise, you will have to drink even more. Remember that two-thirds of our bodies consists of water and we are dependent on it for healthy bodily function.

Water assists the body's cooling system, aids digestion, removes toxins and helps to keep our joints mobile and supple. Water can also improve the texture of the skin. You may need to discipline yourself to drink enough water – as a starter, it is a good idea to put at least a litre of water in the fridge every morning to be drunk by the end of the day. Ideally, use filtered or bottled water, or tap water in a filter jug. If you work during the day, then keep a bottle of water by you throughout the day. Water can dull your appetite and will keep those hunger pangs at bay if you want to maintain your weight – or lose a little.

Balancing act

Most doctors, nutritionists and dieticians will recommend that you eat a balanced diet and developing this balance in your mind will help you to eat both healthily and enjoyably – after all, eating should be one of life's greatest pleasures. We know that the body requires some foods more than others and you should be able to accommodate this easily and efficiently without even thinking about it.

There are several ways to illustrate a typical nutritionally balanced diet. You can imagine it as a pie divided into portions showing the ratio of portions required on a daily basis, or a food pyramid, which shows the larger sections of food group at the bottom, and the smallest required portions at the top. Basically, they both illustrate that the largest proportion of our food should be complex carbohydrates, followed by fruit and vegetables. Protein and dairy products come next, with fats and sugar featuring at the tip of the pyramid or the smallest section of the pie – to be used sparingly, if at all.

So if you apply this to your own dinner plate when you sit down for a meal, you should imagine two-fifths being carbohydrates, such as rice, pasta, potatoes, etc., two-fifths vegetables or salad, and one-fifth protein (meat, fish, cheese, eggs, etc.)

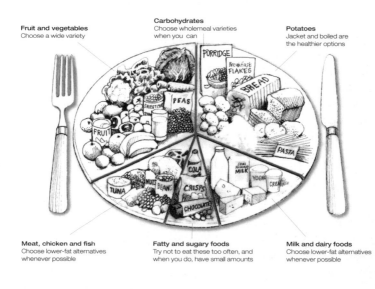

Fruit and vegetables
Choose a wide variety

Carbohydrates
Choose wholemeal varieties when you can

Potatoes
Jacket and boiled are the healthier options

Meat, chicken and fish
Choose lower-fat alternatives whenever possible

Fatty and sugary foods
Try not to eat these too often, and when you do, have small amounts

Milk and dairy foods
Choose lower-fat alternatives whenever possible

Complex carbohydrates

As already outlined, the highest intake or number of servings every day should come from complex carbohydrate foods, preferably unrefined. These include wholemeal varieties of bread, cereals, pasta, brown rice and jacket potatoes. It is worth bearing in mind that these foods are best eaten without butter or fat-rich sauces, as it is these 'extras' that pile on the calories and offer few nutrients. Also it is worth noting that refined carbohydrates such as white bread, white rice and ordinary pasta contain more sugar and will not help with weight loss or weight maintenance regime. The same applies to the added fat to be found in fried (sautéed) and roasted potatoes, so go for baked oven chips (fries) and jacket potatoes – these are the healthier options, along with boiled potatoes.

Fruit and vegetables

Fruit and vegetables more or less have equal billing with complex carbohydrates, and it may be easier to think of your combined daily intake of both of these groups as six or seven portions. A portion is what you would consider a normal serving – the proportion being more important to the overall balance. Lengthy cooking times will reduce nutrient value, so try to eat some raw or lightly cooked vegetables in this mix.

Protein

Both meat and dairy products are important sources of protein and you should eat around two portions of each every day. Bear in mind that many meats, cheeses and some yoghurts are high in fat, so always try to eat the low-fat versions and as already suggested, remove fat from meat and skin from poultry. Remember, as a general rule, the harder the cheese the more fat it contains. So go easy on the Parmesan!

The extras

The higher the fat or refined sugar content of food, the less you need in your healthy balanced diet, so these should make up the smallest proportions of the pyramid or pie. Okay, a little bit of what you fancy does you good – but in moderation, so that it remains only as an occasional special treat.

What's healthy and what's not

Although advice on healthy eating encourages us to take more care with our diet, some people are still confused as to which foods are unhealthy, including fats, specific nutrients, carbohydrates, sugars, alcohol and antioxidants. The media is also full of messages about possible dangers from additives during food manufacture and the potentially harmful chemicals used for crop growth and protection.

The list below gives further information on some of the food areas and subjects that may affect you on a daily basis. They are in alphabetical order, and not in any particular order of merit.

Alcohol

Alcohol is thought to be good for you – but only if taken in moderation. It can raise the levels of high-density lipoproteins (HDLs), which lower cholesterol in the blood. Also the tannins in red wine are thought to slow the oxidation of HDLs, which is a further benefit to the cardiovascular system. The official recommended weekly intake of alcoholic drinks is up to 28 units for men and 21 units for women. A unit is 8 grams (10 ml) – roughly equivalent to a 125 ml glass of wine, half a pint of beer or a single measure of spirit. These guidelines are given for health reasons but alcohol intake also has an effect on your weight. So, if you do cut down on alcohol, you will be healthier and lose weight at the same time!

Excessive alcohol is like sugar water – it can be quickly stored in the form of fat – and should be avoided. A good way to keep your levels down is to drink alcohol only when you are eating. This way the drink is metabolised at a slower rate and combines with other foods producing fewer fat reserves. If cutting down is easier to do than completely stopping, then do so. Just try it for one month to see and feel the positive effects. Try halve your alcoholic intake or, perhaps, have an alcohol-free day three times a week. A good tip is to drink water to quench your thirst, and then sip your tipple for the taste and pleasure.

Allergies

Although not related specifically to our healthy diet, many people do suffer allergic reactions to certain types of food and drink, possibly without ever realising it. So balancing your food intake and eating more complex carbohydrates could influence your well-being in more ways than one. For example, people who suffer from irritable bowel syndrome (IBS) may find that cutting out wheat, rye, barley and oats will reduce their gluten intake, which is a main cause of the problem.

This is where your food diary (see page 48) will be useful. While keeping a record of what you eat, it may be worth recording any incidence of existing health problems that you already have – headaches, migraines, insomnia, tummy upsets, indigestion, wind, etc. Then you can see if following a healthier diet helps you reduce their occurrence – it may also reduce your weight. Interestingly, it can sometimes be the foods that you crave the most that can cause your allergy problems. If you suspect that you have an allergic reaction to a certain food or drink, visit a nutritionist to help you identify the specific cause (see Chapter 10 – Natural Therapies).

Caffeine

Large doses of caffeine are not recommended, being linked to an increased risk of high blood pressure as previously outlined. Caffeine can also stimulate the release of insulin, causing your blood sugar to drop, making you feel hungry. Caffeine is addictive and the first step is to try to cut down on your caffeine intake, and the first move is to simply drink decaffeinated tea and coffee. Also bear in mind that there is probably more caffeine in strong tea than a weak coffee! Try to cut down on both, if you are drinking throughout the day, and perhaps introduce other hot drinks such as herbal tea. Think about drinking water with your meals instead of coffee or tea. Certainly avoid colas and fizzy drinks, which will probably contain both caffeine and sugar.

Cholesterol

Despite its recently acquired reputation as a dangerous substance, cholesterol is an essential part of our body make-up and is only dangerous when there is too much of it. There are two types. High-density lipoprotein (HDL) cholesterol plays an important role for digestion, stress and bone development. Low density lipoprotein (LDL) cholesterol is more dangerous. If found in excess, it can stiffen or stick to the artery walls and narrow the blood vessels.

You can boost your HDL cholesterol by avoiding food containing saturated fats and by eating plenty of fish, pulses, fruits and vegetables, and even taking a regular glass of red wine. LDL cholesterol comes from saturated fats in meat, lard (shortening), some cooking oils and dairy products, so remove fat and skin from meat and try to cut down on butter, cream, etc. Olive oil is the best choice for salad dressings and cooking. Eggs have been listed for years as high in cholesterol but recent research shows them not to be particularly high in saturated fats. However, you should not have more than one or two per week. Have your cholesterol reading checked once a year, especially if there is a history of high cholesterol in the family. Eat plenty of oily fish, which contain omega-3 (essential fatty acids), associated with decreasing the risk of heart disease. See also Fats, Fish oil and Garlic in this section.

Cooking methods

The way a food is cooked can make the difference between healthy and unhealthy eating. As a general rule, poach, boil or grill (broil) your food rather

A little of what you fancy ...

Every year I play golf in Devon and what I look forward to, apart from the golf and the breathtaking views of Dartmoor, is a Devon cream tea. Although I suppose I could could eat these at any time, waiting a whole year to sample this one indulgent tea-time treat makes it pure heaven.

I'm not one for cakes and sweet things, so it is no hardship for me to avoid these on a day-to-day basis – except when I go to France on holiday, when the aroma of freshly baked baguettes and croissants tempts me to change my breakfast eating habits for a week or so. But like the cream tea, the real treat is having them occasionally – having them whenever I liked wouldn't have the same effect. (And anyway, the swimming and extra games of tennis while on holiday help to ease the calories away again ...)

than deep-frying, frying (sautéing) and roasting. Hot stir-frying, microwaving, steaming and pressure cooking are also healthy alternatives. If you do need to cook in fat, avoid the use of standard cooking oils and lard (shortening) – use olive oil.

A wok can be used for many different types of healthy stir-fries. Use a minimum of oil and cook hot and fast, stirring all the time. Make sure the vegetables stay firm and crispy to retain maximum flavour and vitamins. If you really need your regular fix of chips (fries), then go for the low-fat, oven-bake variety.

If you fancy a change from steamed or boiled vegetables, try roasting them in a hot oven. The baking will caramelise the natural sugars and create a very distinctive flavour. Cut the vegetables into strips and lay individually, before lightly spraying with olive oil to prevent them drying up. If you are looking for an alternative to those fat-laden roasted potatoes, cut up potatoes, par-boil, brush very lightly with olive oil and grill. Delicious!

Dairy foods

Dairy foods will supply calcium, protein and vitamins A and B12. However, many have a high fat content. Saturated fat (see Cholesterol, page 56) should be avoided, so it is best to keep to skimmed or semi-skimmed milk, low-fat yoghurts and low-fat cheeses. As a general rule, the harder the cheese, the more saturated fat it is likely to contain. Try and keep to this plan on an everyday basis and then enjoy those special treats occasionally. Try low-fat crème fraîche or ice cream as a good alternative to single (light) or double (heavy) cream to accompany those delicious strawberries. (Do check the sugar content, however, especially if you are trying to watch your weight – it is often surprisingly high, making these low-fat products very high in calories.) Don't be tempted to cut out all dairy products. If you do, this will affect your calcium and mineral intake. Instead, just keep to the low-fat variety and if you suspect there may be any shortfall in your diet, consider taking calcium and mineral supplements (see Chapter 5 – Vitamins and Minerals).

Digestion

Some people take indigestion tablets on a regular basis, especially at night. This should not be necessary, and can often be avoided by changing bad eating or drinking habits. Older men in particular can suffer from indigestion for years and simply think that it is normal. It isn't, and it is likely that anyone changing to a healthy diet will reduce their indigestion symptoms within days, possibly for ever. Drinking alcohol and eating late at night is not good news for indigestion sufferers – so don't do it.

Digestion takes place in two stages, both of which are relevant to our diet. First, the mechanical process of chewing, which we all tend to do quite badly. The pace of modern-day life may see us grabbing food quickly and eating on the run. But even when we sit down to dinner sometimes our attention is more on the television rather than our food. So, draw a deep breath, and think about chewing and tasting when you eat. Make your meals last longer – and enjoy the experience. This different approach will make your meals taste far better and will prepare your food for the second phase of digestion in the stomach, when your gastric juices will start the metabolic transformation of your food. This restores the natural balance of acidity and alkalinity in the stomach, at the same time helping the body to absorb more nutrients, and is also the first major step in ridding yourself of any indigestion. A bonus of eating slowly is that your brain will register that full-up feeling after around 20 minutes – before you go for those second helpings or tempting desserts. So you can throw those indigestion tablets away after a couple of weeks.

Drinks

I have already advocated drinking plenty of water (at least six glasses every day), preferably still. To make the water more interesting, experiment by adding a little natural fruit juice. Read labels on drinks very carefully and avoid sugar and additives, which will mean cutting out colas and equivalents. Remember that low-calorie drinks are not calorie-free, just lower than normal – which was high to begin with.

Drink wine with your meal rather than beer or spirits and sip only when you are eating. Sports drinks will just give you more sugar, so drink water and eat a banana for a better (and cheaper) energy-boost.

Eggs

We know that eggs are good for you, and they are the most versatile of foods to conjure up quick meals – omelettes, scrambled, poached, hard-boiled (hard-cooked), etc. They are low in calories and contain very high protein, as well as many important vitamins and minerals, including iron, calcium and vitamins A, B, C and D. Many doctors are wary of eggs (particularly the yolks) because of their high cholesterol rating (215 milligrams against the recommended intake of 300 milligrams a day). However, recent research indicates that unhealthy levels of cholesterol are influenced by saturated fats, which is not found in eggs. If you suffer from high cholesterol, then obviously watch your egg intake. Eating old or cracked eggs is also dangerous, so check the sell-by dates very carefully and always store them in your refrigerator. A simple test of an egg's freshness is to place it in a bowl of water. Fresh eggs sink to the bottom while stale eggs float rounded-end up, as the air pocket increases with age. Never give raw eggs (for example in home-made mayonnaise) to pregnant women, babies, children or elderly people, because of the risk of salmonella poisoning. Egg whites contain hardly any cholesterol or saturated fat so egg white beaten and included in desserts can provide a good alternative if you are watching your weight.

Fish oil

Despite what we hear about the healthy aspects of a low-fat diet, there are some fats that are actually good for us (see Fats, page 50) and eating fish regularly will help to provide them. Sea fish feature a high iodine content and B-vitamins are found in all fish. Oily fish are valuable sources of vitamins A, D and E, together with the omega-3 essential fatty acids. Omega-3, which helps to promote healthy blood flow and is also known to reduce some heart palpitations, can be taken conveniently in supplement form but you can get enough naturally by eating fish at least two or three times a week. Omega-3 is contained in sardines, mackerel, herring, trout, salmon, tuna, pilchards, kippers and sprats, as well as flax and pumpkin seeds, so you have no excuses. Cod liver oil is an excellent source of omega-3s and also contains vitamins A and D. Some research also shows that omega-3 can reduce inflammation in arthritic joints.

Fruit

Fruit can be your salvation when hunger pangs start to show themselves in the afternoon or at suppertime (especially if trying to lose weight). Eat what you like, but bear in mind a little word of caution: apart from breakfast, fruit should not be eaten at meal times. You may well ask what harm there may be in a simple fruit salad after a meal? The answer is that fruit mixed with other food will be delayed in the digestive process, fermenting and losing some of its nutritional value. So, ideally, eat fruit an hour or two before or after a meal, when it will do the most good.

After washing thoroughly, eat the fruit with the skin. This provides fibre, which increases the vitamin value. It also lowers the glycaemic index of the food (see page 65), which decreases the amount of blood glucose released into the system. This is especially useful for people with diabetes, and those who want to keep an eye on their weight. The old saying: 'An apple a day keeps the doctor away' has been proved correct by recent research, which shows that by eating two apples a day cholesterol levels can be lowered by up to ten per cent.

Bear in mind that the beloved tomato is really a fruit, and recognised as an excellent source of nutrients. Eat lots of them – best fresh, but puréed or even canned are nearly as good, so have whichever you prefer.

Fruit juice

Do not presume that all commercial fruit juice is full of goodness and vitamins. Real fruit is better than commercial juice, and home-made juice is best of all because the pulp contains lots of fibre. We are all busy people and it is certainly a luxury to make your own juice – but always worth it. Bear in mind that fruit juice, like fruit, is a complex carbohydrate so you should drink water with your meals, not fruit juice. If you purchase fruit juice, read the labels carefully, checking the sugar content. Go for the most natural variety you can afford. Note that juice has a higher glycaemic index (GI) than the fruit it comes from. Apple and tomato juice have a lower GI than orange juice. Avoid sweet juices with a high GI such as pineapple or grape juice.

Garlic

Did you know that garlic was used extensively as an antiseptic for wounded soldiers in the First World War? Certainly one of nature's healers, garlic is recommended for both internal and external use for just about every ailment invented. Research shows that garlic can help to reduce heart disease by lowering blood cholesterol and a DAS compound (dialkyl disulphide) found in garlic can affect the growth of cancer cells in the colon, lung and skin. Garlic is also said to have a positive effect on the immune system (see Chapter 9). It is an ingredient that should be included regularly in your diet.

You can store peeled garlic cloves in a jar covered with olive oil in the fridge and they will last for weeks. Then use the garlic-flavoured oil for sautéing, stir-frying and salads. Garlic supplements are plentiful, but check the contents carefully as some contain more garlic than others, and many are manufactured to be odourless. A cheap source of garlic is garlic powder, which can be used as seasoning when cooking – it is readily available from your local supermarket.

Milk

Milk is good for you, supplying a rich source of calcium, protein and vitamins. However, it contains saturated fat, and it may trigger eczema, catarrh or asthma (goat's milk can be a good alternative in some allergy cases). Ideally go for skimmed milk, or if you find this too watery, use semi-skimmed as a compromise. After a while, your tastebuds will adjust and full-cream milk will taste like double-fat cream! Normal milk contains around 4 per cent fat, semi-skimmed about 1.7 per cent, and fully-skimmed milk zero fat. With all dairy products, it is important to keep them in your diet (a couple of servings a day or supplement equivalent) but always try to keep to the low-fat variety. If you are allergic to normal milk or dairy products you can always try soya milk which, although slightly more expensive, is a very good substitute. Also remember that cream is full of fat and it's worth whipping some single cream rather than using double (heavy) cream, or buy a small milk frother to pump your semi-skimmed milk into something resembling cream!

Pasta

Pasta is a carbohydrate that supplies fibre, starch, proteins, vitamins and minerals. The problem is that it can also add pounds to your waistline. Ideally go for wholewheat pasta, which is a more healthy, unrefined form. Pasta should be on the banned list along with white bread if you are trying to shed a few pounds. Bought pasta will probably be made from bleached flour with the addition of butter, eggs, cheese, oils, etc. Nothing can beat the taste of home-made and it is so simple to make using wholemeal flour and eggs, especially with a simple pasta machine to help you create your favourite shapes. But remember, it is also what you put on the pasta that can add those inches around the waist. Pasta addicts should try natural wholewheat pasta with olive oil and garlic (*aglio e olio*) or olive oil, garlic and fresh mixed herbs (*spaghetti alle erbe*). Reduce your intake of meat and cheese sauces.

Potatoes

Many nutritionists that I know recommend the potato as an excellent source of energy, folic acid and vitamin C, although many of its nutritive values are lost when it is actually peeled and cooked. It is not a 'slow' sugar as some experts describe, as its glycaemic index rating changes when cooked, especially when baked or fried (sautéed). Add cooking oil or lard (shortening) to your baked potatoes or chips (fries) and you have a sure-fire recipe for weight gain. Jacket potatoes are an ideal meal, especially with salad or vegetables. Be careful and think about what you pile on top though.

Rice

Processed (white) rice is refined to a degree that removes most of the vitamins and minerals, and it is usually the only rice available when eating out. Brown rice is a healthier alternative as it still has the bran and germ attached, has a much higher fibre content, and retains most of its vitamins and minerals. The downside is that brown rice takes longer to cook and is slightly more chewy (but very tasty). Whichever you eat, the healthier option is always to go for boiled rice rather than fried. Left-over rice should always be cooled quickly and then stored in the fridge. When reheating, make certain it is piping hot all the way through. If you are keen on curries, then learn to cook your own with fresh herbs and spices, but without the butter or ghee that most recipes use.

Salads

Salads are an important part of any healthy diet, but do not be alarmed. I'm not talking about a few limp lettuce leaves with half a tomato and a bit of cucumber and celery. Please forget anything like that pathetic excuse for a salad. Instead, try mixing and matching all your favourite raw salad ingredients and vegetables (lightly cooked, if you prefer) – and do be adventurous. Remember, you can eat as much as you like without putting on weight, and any left-overs always make useful snacks before lunch or dinner.

Try lettuce (there are dozens of varieties to choose from), cabbage, broccoli, cauliflower, spinach, beansprouts, (bell) peppers, garlic, raw mushrooms, onions, radishes, cucumber, celery, cheese, carrots, nuts, tomatoes, sugar snap peas, mangetout (snow peas), French (green) beans, peas, hard-boiled (hard-cooked) eggs, cooked diced bacon, tuna, anchovies, courgettes (zucchini), apple, grapes, avocado, chicken, prawns (shrimp), crab, salmon, ham, asparagus, etc. All full of nutrition. And don't forget to add some simple dressings to bring out the taste. Put three parts olive oil to two parts red wine vinegar in a screw-topped jar with a small spoonful of mustard, a pressed garlic clove, low-fat mayonnaise and a little crème fraîche. Give a shake and enjoy!

How you present your salad can make all the difference. Grate or slice most of the ingredients into different shapes. Choose colours that complement each other and toss them together with dressing. Instead of slicing hard boiled (hard-cooked) eggs and placing on salad, try chopping them up very finely and sprinkling over the top.

Salt

We all probably eat too much salt (sodium), because most processed foods contain it, and most restaurant kitchens over use it – including celebrity chefs on TV. Salt is associated with high blood pressure and hypertension, especially as we get older or are overweight. Salt can also create water retention, which many women experience. If you stop adding any salt to your food, you will be a lot healthier and will still receive more than your fair share of sodium quite naturally. Instead of salt you can use healthier flavour-enhancers such as lemon, Tabasco or fresh herbs. If you must have salt on your food, try adding only a minute amount at the cooking stage rather than at the dinner table – or you can buy low-sodium alternatives. Take-away food contains loads of fat, sugar and salt, so don't go adding even more when you get home. If you do suffer from high blood pressure, your doctor will advise removing salt from your diet, so you will have to read your food labels very carefully. You should try to avoid foods with more than 0.2 gram of sodium per 100 grams – and it may astound you to learn that cornflakes contain five times that amount!

Snacks

Many of us actually think that we don't snack between meals, but we do! (Just check that food diary.) If you are one of those people who say, 'I only have to look at a biscuit and I put on weight', the chances are that you don't just look at it – you eat it! Most of us eat far more than we realise during the course of a day. But you don't have to give up snacking between meals, just take more care about what the snacks contain. If you need to snack, choose food items that will be good for you. Keep on hand a good supply of fruit, nuts and seeds and always have a store of ready-to-eat raw vegetables in the fridge, such as carrot sticks, cucumber sticks, cauliflower florets or wedges of red, green and yellow (bell) peppers. You can use natural yoghurt (with a touch of garlic if you like) or a cottage cheese as a vegetable dip. Delicious!

You can even polish off a bowl of wholegrain cereal with semi-skimmed milk as a late breakfast. And don't forget the fruit. Make it a little more interesting by cutting it into bite-size chunks. Treat yourself to new foods and make them interesting and special – it will make all the difference to the way you feel.

Sugar

Sugar (or glucose) is associated with heart disease, diabetes, obesity and tooth decay. It is also addictive because of its effect on energy levels and moods. We all need sugar but we do not need to add much sugar to our food as it will be naturally produced by the body from a balanced diet. Manufactured sugar in sweets (candies), chocolate, cakes, etc. will give your body a high-energy fix and then release too much insulin as a reaction to curb the excess energy. Your blood sugar then drops to a low again and the uneven cycle begins. This is not taking into account the amount of 'empty' calories that are being piled into your body at the same time. Ideally, we need to eat little and often to maintain a steady glucose level, which will then be released by the body from stored fats as and when it needs it. If you have a sweet tooth, you can always use a sugar substitute as a temporary measure, with a view to reducing its use over the following weeks or months. The first step is to cut down the sugar you add to your food. If you take sugar in hot drinks, take one sugar instead of two, or half a spoonful instead of one, and so on.

Vegetables

Most 50-year-olds will have heard their mother say, 'Eat your greens' because they were in short supply after the war – and she knew they were good for you. Fruits, vegetables, herbs and cereals should be the mainstay of our diet and we have to ensure that our eating habits develop around them. Raw vegetables are at their nutritional best, as the longer you cook a vegetable the more vitamins are wasted. So go for lightly cooked vegetables (see page 56, Cooking methods), cooking quickly and retaining that 'crunchy' taste. Use as little liquid as possible. Then use the same liquid to cook other vegetables or to make a soup or gravy to retain all those nutrients. There will be no cooking problem with salad ingredients as they will probably be raw anyway. Remember that a healthy diet requires you to eat a minimum of at least five fruit or vegetable portions every day. Buy fruit and vegetables that are as fresh as possible as vitamins will diminish with age and storage. Fresh vegetables are better than frozen, but frozen vegetables are still better than old vegetables. Best of all, choose fresh, whole vegetables that are organically grown.

Wine

As already discussed, when it comes to drinking alcohol, moderation is the order of the day. Many health experts agree that a little of what you fancy does you good when it comes to beer and wine, but wine has an advantage when drinking with a meal. A moderate amount of red wine can be of benefit to the blood, helping to reduce both cholesterol and clotting. But alcohol carries many calories and has a high glycaemic index rating (see below), so releasing sugar into the blood very quickly. Drinking only when eating will slow this process down. Never drink wine when you are thirsty. Drink water to quench your thirst and then have some wine with your meal. Just a couple of glasses a day with your meals will be good for you and will not add extra weight. Of course, if you drink less wine, then you can afford to treat yourself to the very best. You could even have a bottle of bubbly every month to celebrate the success of your healthier diet.

Glycaemic index

The glycaemic index (GI) is used to measure a particular food in relation to its effect on raising sugar in the blood. This system was developed to aid diabetics and help prevent high blood-sugar levels (hyperglycaemia) when choosing foods. Carbohydrates with a high GI rating cause a high level of blood-sugar. Complex carbohydrates, which are absorbed more slowly, produce a gradual and prolonged sugar rise, providing sustained energy throughout the day. A poor diet full of processed food or sugar-related items will result in higher blood-sugar levels and high insulin levels, one of the main factors responsible for the development of obesity, high cholesterol and diabetes. So take heed. Foods with a lower GI tend to contain more fibre and so are also more likely to fill you up for longer. I list some of the popular foods with their higher and lower GI readings below. Some of the food items may surprise you.

Higher GI rating

alcohol	honey
bananas	ice cream
bread, white	jams (conserves)
biscuits (cookies)	jellies (clear conserves)
doughnuts	melon
cakes	pasta, ordinary
carrots, cooked	pineapple
cereals with sugar	pizza
chocolate	potatoes
cornflakes	quiche
cornflour (cornstarch)	rice, white
glucose	sugar
hamburgers	sweets (candies)

Lower GI rating

apples	grapefruit
artichokes	lentils
bamboo shoots	lettuce
bread, wholemeal	mushrooms
broccoli	oranges
brussels sprouts	pasta, wholemeal
cabbage	pears
carrots, raw	(bell) peppers
cauliflower	radishes
celery	rice, brown
courgettes (zucchini)	soya beans
cucumbers	spinach
French (green) beans	tomatoes

Food labelling

All food labels now have to contain certain elements of statutory information. These are the actual name of the product, the manufacturer's name and address, a list of ingredients in descending order of weight, and a 'use by' or 'best before' date. 'Use by' dates are used on perishable foods that need to be eaten before the designated date to avoid the possibility of food poisoning. 'Best before' dates are used on less perishable foods that will lose their eating quality but would not actually be harmful if eaten after the expiry date.

Where food labelling is less clear is in the area of nutrition information and claims. Nutritional labelling is still only optional unless a nutrition claim is made (e.g. high-fibre, low-salt) but most manufacturers do give at least the basic information on how much energy (calories), protein, carbohydrate and fat a food contains per 100 g and sometimes, more helpfully, per portion. Some labels also give additional information on saturates, sugars, fibre, sodium, vitamins, minerals, etc., but the problem is that the information is sometimes in a complicated and unhelpful format.

Food labelling does have its plus points. At least we get good information on how to store and cook foods, and when to eat them by. Many large supermarkets also now try to give helpful 'healthy eating' information and logos on packs to facilitate more nutritious choices. But a succession of food scares (salmonella, BSE, pesticide residues, etc.) has left us rightly suspicious about the food we eat, and consumers now want to know more about the food that they buy.

As yet, current food labelling means that consumers do not have the right to know whether or not a food is derived from or contains genetically modified

Understanding food labels

Ingredients   Ingredients are listed in descending weight order – the higher up the list, the more there is in the food.

Energy   Checking the energy content on food labels can be very helpful if you are dieting. Energy intake is measured in terms of calories, which is the kcal figure on the label.

Protein   Protein is important for body growth and tissue repair, but most adults in Western societies get more than enough. You won't need to scrutinise the amount on food labels unless you're shopping for a strict vegetarian or an athlete.

Carbohydrate   Carbohydrates provide energy. Starch is a healthy form of carbohydrate, whereas sugars should be eaten in moderation only. If the label only gives one figure for carbohydrate, it is the total for starch and sugars – check the ingredients listing to see if sugars have been added to the food.

Sugars   Some labels also give separate information on sugars. Remember it is advisable to keep your intake down – too many sugars can cause tooth decay, offer little nutrition, and will pile on the weight. However, sugars found in milk and whole fruit (not juice) are an exception – they are tooth-friendly.

Fat   Fat is the most concentrated source of calories. The three main types of fat are saturates, monounsaturates and polyunsaturates. Monounsaturates are the 'healthiest', followed by polyunsaturates and saturates. But fat is fat whichever the type, and you should try to keep your overall intake down.

Saturates   Look for foods low in saturates as well as low in total fat. Eating too many saturates may raise blood cholesterol and increase the risk of heart disease.

Fibre   Fibre is important for a healthy digestive system and regular bowel movement. Check the label to find out where the fibre comes from. It's better to get fibre from foods that naturally contain it – such as wholegrain cereals, fruit and vegetables – rather than from added bran or other refined fibres.

Sodium   Sodium is the part of salt that can raise blood pressure. It is desirable to keep down your intake, especially if you have heart disease in the family.

Vitamins and minerals Some food labels also tell you how much of certain vitamins and minerals are in the product. The figures indicate the percentage of the recommended daily allowance you'll get in a serving or 100 g/4 oz of the food.

products. In the case of soya, even the manufacturers themselves don't know whether their products may contain genetically modified soya or not, because the big American producers are allowed to export mixed batches of standard and genetically modified beans to Europe.

In addition, most fruit and vegetables, except those certified as organic, are likely to have been treated with chemicals. This is not made clear at the point of sale, so you should presume the worst. Remove any outside leaves or skin from fresh produce and scrub very thoroughly any fruit or vegetables where the skin is to be eaten.

Some manufacturers make nutritional claims for their products, but these do not tell the whole story. For example, a reduced-calorie food could still be high in sodium, and a low-fat food may contain large quantities of sugar. Not all the claims are regulated by law either, so remain sceptical.

Low-fat spreads are exempt from the guidelines for low-fat claims. So a 'low-fat' spread could have 40 g/1¾ oz of fat per 100 g/4 oz. That makes it a lot lower in fat than butter or margarine, but it's still a high-fat food relative to others in the diet.

Be aware of hidden fat and sugar. Remember that various types of fat and sugar can occur several times throughout the ingredients list, so just because the first ingredient isn't sugar- or fat-related doesn't necessarily mean it is a healthy food.

Note that any figures referring to vitamins and minerals indicate the percentage of the recommended daily allowance (RDA) that will be found in a normal serving of 100 g/4 oz. See Recommended daily allowances, page 80.

E-numbers are given to food additives approved for use in all EU countries. Both 'natural' and synthetic additives have designated E-numbers. All have to be proved 'safe, effective and necessary' before they are used. Unfortunately, just as we started to get used to E-numbers, the trend is now to bamboozle you with the chemical name instead.

CHAPTER 5

Vitamins and Minerals

The correct supply of micro-nutrients can help us cope with whatever the day has in store.

Without vitamins and minerals, we just would not be able to function. With them, we can run, smile and be healthy for the many years ahead. Vitamins and minerals are essential to our very existence, yet we underestimate the important role they play in our everyday needs.

Vitamins and minerals help us to grow into fit and healthy human beings, give us energy and aid our fight against disease and infection. Thanks to these micronutrients, most of us can get up in the morning ready to tackle another busy day at work or whatever the day will throw at us. Because nearly every micronutrient cannot be manufactured by the body, it has to be obtained from the food that we eat, and sticking to a varied, well-balanced diet should supply more than enough for most of us (see Chapter 4, A Healthy Diet).

The World Health Organisation recommends that everyone should eat at least five portions of fruit and vegetables a day. Unfortunately, the truth is that most of us consume nowhere near this amount – on average, we manage a pathetic three. And because fresh foods start to lose their goodness the moment they are harvested, even those who do won't necessarily be getting as much as they need.

These factors and others – such as stress, alcohol, age and hormonal balance – may mean that many people are not getting anywhere near sufficient levels of nutrients (see the chart on page 80). Also the damage caused by free radicals (see Antioxidants, page 77) can cause havoc in the body and damage long-term health, especially as we reach middle age. For example, a recent study reported in *The Lancet* found that increasing daily intake of vitamin C from fruit and vegetables by just 50 g/2 oz (the equivalent of two pieces of broccoli or fruit) reduced the risk of death from cardiovascular disease, heart attack and cancer.

In our efforts to combat such damage and to ensure maximum intake of vital nutrients, a third of the population are now turning to supplements. Women especially are thought to need extra nutrition at various stages in their lives, while slimmers and vegetarians may also need a little extra help. As we grow older vitamins and minerals play an even more important role in our longevity and health. At the end of this chapter you will find a list of foods that supply particular vitamins or minerals, including the recommended daily allowance for each one.

Vitamins

There are two types of vitamins – fat-soluble and water-soluble. The fat-soluble vitamins, which are A, D and E, can be stored in the body, mainly in the liver. The water-soluble vitamins – all the B-complex vitamins and vitamin C – are excreted through our urine. With the exception of vitamin B12, these cannot be stored in the body.

Upon entering the body, a vitamin travels through the bloodstream to the cells, where it joins up with enzymes to do its job. The cells can only use so much of the vitamin and when a certain ceiling is reached, the vitamin will be excreted or stored. So it is important to remember that there are no benefits to be gained by ingesting huge quantities of extra vitamins. Taking more supplements than your body actually needs can be a complete waste of money.

Vitamin A (retinol)

This particular vitamin is an antioxidant and is essential for top-to-toe health. It promotes growth, strong bones and healthy skin, hair, teeth and gums. It also builds resistance to respiratory diseases and maintains the health of the outer layers of tissues and organs. It only occurs naturally in animal foods, but beta-carotene from vegetable sources can be converted by the body into vitamin A if we run short. Low levels can lead to poor eyesight, skin infections and dry and flaky skin. Vitamin A is sometimes given as a supplement to help treat acne and psoriasis. Good natural sources of vitamin A are eggs, dairy products, liver and fish. Margarine also contains vitamin A, because it is added as a legal requirement during manufacture. Vitamin A can also be found in brightly coloured fruit and vegetables, such as (bell) peppers and carrots.

Beta-carotene

If the body happens to be running low on vitamin A, this nutrient will take over its role. Beta-carotene also has its own important jobs to do – acting as an antioxidant as well as protecting the skin against damage caused by the sun's harmful ultraviolet rays. Because it is one of a family of carotenoids that provide the pigmentation in plants, most fruit and vegetables rich in beta-carotene are vivid shades of orange, green and yellow – broccoli, (bell) peppers, tomatoes, carrots, apricots, peaches and mangoes.

B-group vitamins

The B-vitamins are needed to maintain a healthy immune system. Vitamin B5 helps to build antibodies, assists wound healing and is thought to have a strengthening effect on the skin when it is combined with other antioxidants. This vitamin is found in beef, eggs, pulses, watercress, tomatoes and wholemeal bread. Vitamin B6 is a vital vitamin for cell oxidation, tissue repair and growth and can be found in wheatgerm, bananas, nuts and oily fish.

Vitamin B1 (thiamin)

Essential for digestion, vitamin B1 helps turn carbohydrates into energy. Therefore, the more carbs we eat, the more vitamin B1 we need. This vitamin also promotes growth and aids in the functioning of the nervous system, muscles and heart. It is often taken as a supplement to ease seasickness and may help to relieve post-operative dental pain. A deficiency can produce confusion and memory loss and a severe lack can cause fatigue, stiffness in the leg muscles and breathlessness when exercising. Many breakfast cereals are 'fortified' with thiamin. Pulses, seeds, tomatoes, brown rice and nuts are also good sources. Meat is not generally a good source with the exception of pork and liver. The vitamin is quite unstable and estimates suggest that at least 20 per cent is lost during domestic food preparation.

Vitamin B2 (riboflavin)

Riboflavin is essential for digestion, helping to convert proteins, fats and carbohydrates into energy. It also assists in growth and reproduction and is an important factor in keeping skin, hair and nails healthy. It is thought that it may benefit vision and alleviate eye fatigue. Foods rich in riboflavin include dairy products, meat (especially liver), eggs, salmon, mackerel, tomatoes and green leafy vegetables. A small amount can be found in tea.

Vitamin B3 (niacin)

As well as aiding the digestive system, vitamin B3 helps the nerves to work and a deficiency can lead to confusion and memory loss. It is found mainly in meat, vegetables (especially potatoes) and cereals, and also in coffee and cocoa. Unlike most other vitamins, it is not easily affected by storage or cooking.

Vitamin B5 (pantothenic acid)

This vitamin has many protective and healing properties. It fights infection by building antibodies, helps to prevent fatigue and assists wound healing and plays a vital role in the release of energy from foods into the body, maintaining healthy growth. Main sources are meat, eggs, pulses, watercress, tomatoes, cereals, vegetables and wholemeal bread.

Vitamin B6 (pyridoxine)

Vitamin B6 is essential for converting proteins into energy in the body. It also helps to maintain healthy skin, teeth and gums and can reduce night muscle spasms, leg cramps and hand numbness. Because it is a natural diuretic, it can help to relieve water retention just before menstruation. It can alleviate nausea, morning sickness and has been recommended for the relief of symptoms associated with pre-menstrual syndrome (PMS). Rich sources are liver, wholegrain cereals, meat and poultry, nuts, bananas and oily fish, such as salmon. Moderate amounts can be found in vegetables such as broccoli, spinach and potatoes. Vitamin B6 is lost during food-processing (heating, canning and freezing), so fresh sources are best.

Vitamin B9 (folic acid or folate)

It is now recommended that pregnant women take regular supplements of folic acid as extra amounts are required for mothers-to-be and natural stores may be inadequate (see page 78, Diets for special needs). In normal use, it can help to ward off anaemia, common symptoms of which are tiredness, forgetfulness and confusion. Folate intake correlates with vitamin C, as many of the sources provide both of these vitamins. Main foods that contribute to total intakes include cereals, beer and vegetables. Most cooking procedures tend to reduce the vitamin, even keeping food hot or reheating. Despite the beer connection, vitamin B9 deficiency may be an indication of an alcohol problem, as alcohol has a negative effect of the absorption of folate.

Vitamin B12 (cobalamin)

This nutrient assists in the formation of red blood cells, thereby preventing anaemia. A brain food, vitamin B12 helps to maintain a healthy nervous system, improving concentration, memory and balance. It also promotes growth and helps to boost energy levels. The body tends to absorb and store this valuable vitamin. A severe deficiency, which would be rare and occur after a long period due to the body's storage, can result in anaemia or brain damage. For humans the only dietary sources of vitamin B12 are animal foods. Richest sources are animal livers, where the vitamin is stored. Meat, eggs and dairy products contain smaller concentrations. It is therefore recommended that vegans, who exclude all animal foods from their diet, should take a vitamin B12 supplement. Also excessive amounts of vitamin C can interfere with Vitamin B12, making it inactive.

Biotin (B group)
This is not a true vitamin but a water-soluble coenzyme that works with the B-complex family. Essential for healthy skin and hair, biotin occurs in many foods, such as cereals, eggs, meat and milk. The richest sources are egg yolks, liver, grains and legumes.

Vitamin C (ascorbic acid)
As an antioxidant, studies have shown that large amounts of vitamin C may help protect against some forms of cancer (mouth, oesophagus, stomach and pancreas) and heart disease. It also helps to heal wounds and burns and is essential for normal healthy growth and metabolism. As a supplement, it is mostly taken to fight against colds and flu by boosting the immune system. Various drugs may also increase the need for vitamin C, including cortisone, aspirin and birth control pills.

Most dietary vitamin C is supplied by vegetables and fruit. Only small amounts come from animal sources, mostly from milk. Among the richest fruit sources are blackcurrants, rosehips and kiwi fruit, but it is also found in oranges (and orange juice), mangoes and strawberries. Vegetable sources include green (bell) peppers, broccoli, cauliflower and brussels sprouts. Potatoes also supply vitamin C but it does decline with storage.

Vitamin C is the least stable of vitamins, being readily lost in cooking or processing. Even keeping vegetables hot after cooking will destroy most of the vitamin C within an hour. Vitamin C in fruit is less volatile, although fruit juice will lose its vitamin C content if left to stand in a fridge. The best way to maximise the intake of vitamin C from fruit and vegetables is to consume as many as possible in their natural form.

Vitamin C enhances the body's iron absorption and is thought to detoxify foreign substances in the liver and to boost the immune function of the body. It is also responsible for producing the protein collagen, which supports the skin structure, helps the strengthening of blood capillaries and prevents bruising. Deficiency of vitamin C is commonly found in elderly people (generally as a result of poor diet) and alcoholics. Heavy smokers may also have poorer absorption and need to take more vitamin C to combat the free radicals generated by smoking.

Vitamin D ————————————————————————————

Vitamin D helps the body utilise calcium and phosphorus to build strong teeth and bones. It is especially important for helping to combat osteoporosis, which is common in post-menopausal women. It is sometimes known as the 'sunshine supplement' because it is actually produced by the action of daylight on the skin and once absorbed in the summer, it can be retained in the body for the winter. Therefore, people who spend most of the day indoors throughout the year or wear all-over clothing may need a vitamin D supplement. It can also be used in the treatment of conjunctivitis, an eye infection. There are few other sources apart from butter, margarine, eggs, milk, oily fish and liver. Some foods may be fortified with vitamin D, for example breakfast cereals, bedtime drinks and yoghurts. Fish oil supplements are a rich source of vitamin D and may be taken by people to help with rheumatism and joint pains.

Vitamin E ————————————————————————————

This vitamin is a powerful antioxidant that looks after the health of the heart and circulation, nerves, muscles and red blood cells. Research has proved that it is essential in the prevention of heart disease. Studying 2,000 patients with heart disease, UK scientists at Cambridge University showed how high doses of vitamin E reduced the risk of both fatal and non-fatal heart attacks by 47 per cent. Scientists at Harvard Medical School in the US believe that the vitamin's antioxidant qualities help to reduce the risk of developing Parkinson's disease. It also works with vitamin A to protect the lungs against air pollution and is thought to protect against skin damage caused by free radicals – studies have shown that a shortage of vitamin E can lead to early ageing of skin cells. Among plant foods, vegetable oils are the most important sources. In addition, it is found in green leafy vegetables and many fruits and nuts. Some breakfast cereals may be fortified with vitamin E, but always check the label. Small amounts do exist in poultry, fish and eggs.

Some experts have claimed that megadoses of vitamin E can improve sports performance, slow down the ageing process, improve sexual libido and prolong cardiac function, although there is little evidence to substantiate any of these claims. But without doubt the vitamin plays an important role in compensating for the action of free radicals in our environment. Research on cancer, heart disease and Parkinson's disease suggest that fewer cases may occur with adequate vitamin E status. So it is well worth ensuring that this vitamin forms an important part of your diet through food or by supplement. There is no evidence of any harm being caused by taking too much of vitamin E.

Minerals

Minerals comprise approximately 6 per cent of our body weight and form the greater proportion of our bones and teeth. A balanced diet that contains a variety of meat, fish, dairy products, nuts, cereals, vegetables and fruit will supply all the minerals we need, which are vital for our well-being. There are three groups – macrominerals, microminerals and trace elements. Macrominerals are required in larger amounts and include calcium, sodium and magnesium. Microminerals are needed in less amounts and include iron, manganese and zinc. Trace elements such as iodine are required in only tiny amounts but even these are necessary.

Calcium

Essential for both developing and maintaining strong healthy bones and teeth, calcium is the most abundant mineral in the human body. However, between the ages of 18 and 35, people reach their maximum bone mass and after this time, calcium levels are depleted from our bodies faster than they are replaced. This happens earlier and more rapidly in women at the time of the menopause, leading to possible loss of bone mass and density (see Chapter 8, Good Health). The main dietary sources are milk and other dairy products. Vegetarians who do not include dairy products in their diet should substitute tofu and calcium-enriched soya milk in order to get the calcium their bodies need. Green leafy vegetables, especially spinach and broccoli, contain substantial amounts, as do sardines, figs, nuts, parsley and watercress.

Chromium

Involved in the production of the hormone insulin, which helps to regulate blood-sugar levels, chromium is often taken as a supplement by people who crave sugary foods. However, insulin-dependent diabetics should not take chromium in supplement form unless advised by their doctor, because it may reduce the body's need for insulin. Chromium has been shown to help lower cholesterol levels. Richest sources are spices, brewer's yeast, meats, whole grains, legumes and nuts.

Copper

Copper aids the creation of the pigment melanin, which helps to protect the skin from the environment. It is found in nuts, lentils, liver and shellfish.

Iodine

Iodine is converted by the body to a substance called iodide. This is needed for the production of the thyroid hormones that regulate metabolic rate – the speed at which oxygen is burned in the body to release energy. As a supplement, iodine may stimulate an under-active thyroid gland, although high levels should not be taken to treat thyroid problems unless under medical supervision. The main source in the UK is milk, as a result of increased use of cattle-feed supplements that contain iodine. It is also to be found in fish, particularly haddock, whiting and herring.

Iron

Important for the formation of red blood cells, iron also delivers oxygen to body tissues to provide energy and general well-being. Iron is lost through bleeding and women can lose a significant amount during menstruation. Deficiency can lead to anaemia, symptoms of which include fatigue, loss of appetite, pallor and light-headedness. The nails may also become brittle. Iron occurs in the diet in two forms, haem iron, which can be found in meat and fish and non-haem iron, which is in legumes and green vegetables. White bread flour and many cereals are fortified with iron, which accounts for the majority of much of the daily intake of people in the Western world.

Magnesium

Magnesium, along with calcium and phosphorus, provides the body's bone structure and strength. It is important for energy release and the functioning of nerves and muscles, as well as promoting a healthier cardiovascular system. Absorption of magnesium occurs in the small intestine and appears to be more efficient when intakes are low. Absorption is also improved by the presence of vitamin D. As a supplement, magnesium is used to alleviate depression and indigestion. Food sources include fish, chicken, wholegrain cereals, nuts, legumes, fish, shellfish, pasta, soya beans, coffee, tea, cocoa and chocolate.

Manganese

Manganese is necessary for the construction of the connective tissue that supports the skin and protects cells from harmful free radicals. The best sources are wholegrains, green leafy vegetables, wholemeal bread and avocados.

Phosphorus

Phosphorus is necessary for maintaining strong healthy bones and teeth. It is also a component of the coenzyme ATP (adenosine triphosphate, for those of you who like to know these things) – the immediate source of energy in muscle tissue. Because it is a stable mineral and contained in most foods, including meat, poultry, fish, eggs, dairy products, cereals, nuts and legumes, deficiency is unlikely, so it is rarely needed as a single supplement.

Selenium

An antioxidant mineral, selenium helps protect the delicate fatty parts of cells from going rancid and is also needed for healthy liver tissue. It has a mutually beneficial relationship with its fellow antioxidant vitamin E, with each enhancing the function of the other. Rich sources include fish and shellfish, offal, red kidney beans, nuts, bread, kidney, lentils, pork, rabbit, veal, dairy products, fruit and vegetables.

Sulphur

Sulphur is needed to create the protein keratin, which is found in skin cells. The best source foods are kidneys, peas and beans. Apart from related amino acids and vitamins there appears to be no requirement for sulphur in any other form and no deficiency has ever been observed.

Zinc

Needed for healthy reproductive and immune systems, zinc is also required for tissue repair and renewal, and for the maintenance of vision, taste and smell. As a supplement, it can be used to treat skin conditions such as acne and eczema, and may help to reduce wound-healing time after burns or surgery. Particularly good sources are lean meat, shellfish and dairy products. Pulses and whole grains are a moderate source, but more important in vegetarian diets.

Antioxidants

Antioxidants help prevent oxygen reacting with molecules in our body in ways that could cause damage, possibly encouraging some cancers and heart disease. The damage is caused by certain varieties of oxygen molecules known as free radicals, which attempt to 'steal' particles (electrons) from the molecules in our cells. Excess free radicals are caused by environmental factors such as pollution and smoking. Antioxidant nutrients and enzymes can sacrifice their own electrons to the free radicals, thus protecting the body's precious cells. The most important antioxidant nutrients are vitamins A (in the form of beta-carotene), C and E, as well as the mineral selenium. So the message is to include plenty of fruit and vegetables in your everyday diet.

Diets for special needs

A good, balanced, healthy diet should provide the correct amount of vitamins and minerals our bodies need. However, there are some circumstances when extra supplements may be needed. For example, environmental factors, lifestyle and illness can all affect the way in which nutrients are absorbed.

Stress

Everyone to a certain extent is affected by stress but the body's response to prolonged anxiety can deplete certain vitamins and minerals. Overactive adrenal glands can use up vitamin C, so a high-dose supplement can help to replace this antioxidant. Stress also depletes the body of B-vitamins, vital to maintain a healthy nervous system, so a B-complex supplement can be beneficial in reducing anxiety symptoms. It may also be helpful to take magnesium to calm the nerves and a multivitamin/mineral supplement.

People on restricted diets

Anyone who has a restricted diet for any reason may not be getting the right balance of vitamins and minerals from their food. Usually if you are on a restricted diet for medical reasons, your doctor will take this into account and recommend any nutritional supplements you may require. But this group also includes those who have restricted their diets for other reasons. For example, slimmers need to make sure that their reduced diet is still adequately balanced and includes all the necessary nutrients. As there are no vegetable sources of vitamin D or B12, vegetarians and vegans may find it necessary to use supplements. Also iron from plants and cereals is more difficult for the body to absorb so vitamin C may be needed to help the absorption of this mineral. A vegan diet may be low in zinc unless large amounts of wholegrains, lentils, peas, nuts, seeds and peas are eaten.

Smokers and drinkers

We know that smoking and drinking to excess are harmful in many ways but they also use up vital antioxidant nutrients, lowering the immune system and making the body more susceptible to disease (see page 77). Smokers and drinkers may need to increase their intake of vitamin C, beta-carotene and vitamin E, or alternatively use a good all-round antioxidant supplement.

The elderly

As we get older our appetite often decreases and it is sometimes difficult to get the necessary nutrients from diet alone. It is important for the elderly to make sure that they are getting enough antioxidant vitamins to help keep the immune system in operation and to assist circulation. It is also a good idea to supplement vitamin D, calcium and magnesium in the diet to help maintain healthy bones. (See also Chapter 13.)

Menopausal women

During the menopause, a woman's body goes through an immense change (see Chapter 8). The body releases more calcium from the bones, and this can sometimes lead to osteoporosis (brittle bone disease). An increase in calcium in the diet could help to prevent the onset of this disease but it needs to be accompanied by vitamin D to ensure the mineral is adequately absorbed. Other symptoms of the menopause can be eased through the correct diet and possibly supplementation of a multivitamin/mineral with additional vitamin C, ideally well in advance.

Taking supplements

A good well-balanced diet should give you all that you need but you can make your own mind up when reviewing the table following this text. This gives the recommended allowance of important nutrients that we all need to remain healthy, with a reminder of which food provides the particular nutrient. In theory you have no need to take any supplements if you eat a balanced diet and live in a friendly environment. But the chances of that are fairly remote: we have no control over how our food is grown, packed, transported and prepared for sale. Even with organic foods we have to trust the soil that it is grown in or what the label tells us. Then when we get the food into our kitchens we remove many of the nutrients when preparing, cooking or freezing. And then there are the effects of a lifestyle that may include drinking, smoking and little exercise.

So it does make some sense to top up on vitamins and minerals especially in the areas that we feel there may be a gap – vegetarians for example, fussy eaters, dieters, the elderly, etc. A multivitamin and mineral supplement taken once a day is probably good practice for most people, and fish oil or garlic may be of added benefit. My advice would be to choose a good make of supplement (this will certainly not be the cheapest – this is one of those areas where you get what you pay for) and to examine the label carefully against what your particular requirements are. Compare the labels on your breakfast cereals too, as some are fortified with vitamins and minerals. High doses of some vitamins and minerals can be dangerous, although you would have to exceed the RDA many times to give cause for any concern. If you have any doubts about your diet or nutritional intake I would recommend a visit to a good nutritionist to evaluate your personal requirements based on your every day 'honest' diet and lifestyle.

Interestingly, a recent 'heart protection' study by scientists at Oxford University, based on research covering 20,000 people over five years, found that taking the recommended daily allowance of vitamins in pill form offered no more protection against heart disease, stroke or cancers than a well-balanced diet. Another point made was that the quality of vitamins is vital, with many synthetic versions not being as powerful as their organic counterparts.

But nutritionists argue that optimal quantities, which **would** reduce risks of disease, are probably higher than the RDA – from two to ten times as much. They also argue, and I have already mentioned, that the food we eat may be nutritionally impoverished through intensive farming, soil depletion and food processing, not to mention storage. So, if in doubt about your diet, a multivitamin and mineral supplement could be a good idea.

Recommended daily allowances
The recommended daily allowance (RDA), or reference nutritional intake (RNI), of vitamins and minerals has been devised for populations and represents the amount of nutrients required by most individuals to prevent the onset of a deficiency disease. The table on the next pages compares the RDA of essential nutrients with the upper safe level for supplementation, as advised by the Council for Responsible Nutrition (CRN) in its report, *Essential Nutrients in Supplements*. If you are taking supplements, to ensure you're not overdoing things, check the amounts on your labels and use the table as a guide.

Nutrient	Best natural sources	RDA	Max daily amount
mg = milligram (one thousandth of a gram) µg = microgram (one millionth of a gram)			
Vitamin A (Retinol)	Cheese, eggs, butter, watercress, melon, tomatoes, cod liver oil, liver, tuna, red (bell) peppers, oranges	800 µg	2,300 µg
Beta-carotene	Green leafy vegetables, broccoli, carrots, sweet potato, tomatoes, watercress, fruit	N/A	20 mg

Nutrient	Best natural sources	RDA	Max daily amount
Vitamin B1 (thiamin)	Watercress, tomatoes, peas, beans, brown rice, yeast extract, breakfast cereals, peanuts	1.4 mg	100 mg
Vitamin B2 (riboflavin)	Eggs, milk, cheese, mackerel, salmon, tomatoes, green leafy vegetables, cornflakes, oats	1.6 mg	200 mg
Vitamin B3 (niacin)	Meat, poultry, oily fish, yeast extract, bread, potatoes, cheese, milk, tomatoes, breakfast cereals	18 mg	450 mg (nicotinamide) 150 mg (nicotinic acid)

Nicotinamide and nicotinic acid are two versions of vitamin B3. Nicotinic acid is not as safe in large quantities as nicotinamide. Therefore, only one form should be taken, never both.

Nutrient	Best natural sources	RDA	Max daily amount
Vitamin B5 (pantothenic acid)	Beef, pig's liver, eggs, pulses, watercress, tomatoes, wholemeal bread, brown rice, nuts, dried fruit	6 mg	500 mg
Vitamin B6 (pyridoxine)	Pig's liver, wholemeal bread, eggs, watercress, nuts, bananas, brewer's yeast, yeast extract, wheat bran, red (bell) peppers, cabbage, kidney beans	2 mg	200 mg
Vitamin B9 (folic acid)	Green leafy veg, broccoli, cheese, pulses, nuts, bananas oranges, yeast extract	200 µg	400 µg
Vitamin B12 (cobalamin)	Meat, poultry, fish, eggs, cheese, milk, breakfast cereals	1 µg	500 µg
Biotin	Vegetables, pig's liver, cheese, eggs, milk, yoghurt, fish, nuts, melon, oranges, brown rice, wholemeal bread	150 µg	500 µg
Vitamin C	Broccoli, carrots, peas, potatoes, watercress, kiwi fruit, melon, oranges, lemons, blackcurrants, tomatoes, (bell) peppers, bananas, strawberries	60 mg	2,000 mg
Vitamin D	Eggs, milk, cottage cheese, fish	5 µg	10 µg

Nutrient	Best natural sources	RDA	Max daily amount
Vitamin E	Green leafy vegetables, eggs, unrefined sunflower or rapeseed oil, peanuts, wheatgerm, wholemeal bread, bananas, tuna	10 mg	800 mg
Calcium	Dairy produce, eggs, canned fish, green leafy vegetables	800 mg	1,500 mg
Chromium	Egg yolk, molasses, brewer's yeast, beef, cheese, wholemeal bread, potatoes, skimmed milk, bananas	N/A	200 µg
Copper	Meat, poultry, fish, avocado, nuts, pulses, bread, chocolate, beer, cider, mushrooms	N/A	2–10 mg
Iodine	Kelp, fish oils, sea salt, vegetables	150 µg	500 µg
Iron	Beef, pork, offal, liver/kidney, spinach, green leafy vegetables, fortified breakfast cereal, figs, dried apricots, wheatgerm, corned beef, plain (semi-sweet) chocolate	14 mg	15 mg
Magnesium	Shellfish, pasta, peas, soya beans, nuts, brewer's yeast, wholemeal bread, fish, chicken, hard cheese, wholegrain cereals	300 mg	350 mg
Phosphorus	Dairy produce, fish, vegetables, meat, nuts, wholegrains	800 mg	1,500 mg
Selenium	Whole wheat grain, offal, fish, shellfish, nuts, dairy products, fruit and vegetables	N/A	200 µg
Zinc	Hard cheese, shellfish, beef, pork, dairy produce, eggs, green vegetables, cereal, chicken	15 mg	15 mg

CHAPTER 6

Slim and Trim

One of the most effective ways of helping yourself look and feel young is to keep an eye on your weight. Carrying extra weight around is not only energy-sapping, it is also positively bad for your health. This chapter is all about achieving and keeping to your ideal weight.

Since the 1980s the number of obese people in the UK has tripled. And as much as 50 per cent of the adult population is overweight, with 17 per cent of men and 21 per cent of women being classified as obese. Obesity is a major killer in the UK, causing more than 30,000 deaths a year. The most worrying statistic is the number of obese children, which has doubled since the 1980s. As many as 10 per cent of six-year-olds are now clinically obese. This is an epidemic! Strangest of all, bread consumption is a third of what it was some 50 years ago, and we eat half as many potatoes and half as much butter. Clearly, something has happened to our eating habits.

Just 50 years ago the average woman weighed 8 st 6 lb (118 lb) and her vital statistics (in inches) read something like 33–23–34. Nowadays the average woman weighs 10 st 5 lb (145 lb) and her vitals are 36–32–38. What happened to that waist? Men don't get off that lightly either. Their average waist size was around 30 inches 50 years ago, compared with today's 38.8 inches and the average weight of 11 st (154 lb) is now 12 st 5 lb (173 lb). So something is going wrong. (For those who are fully metricated, that's 53.5 kg and 84–55–86 changing to 65.7 kg and 91–81–97 for the women, and 70 kg and 76 cm changing to 78.5 kg and 99 cm for the men but somehow it doesn't have the same ring to it!)

A healthy diet and exercise routine will help you stay in shape and keep you fit and healthy.

We know that weight gain tends to occur with increasing age, with particular increases in fat occurring between the ages of 30 and 45. In women, increases in body weight may follow pregnancy, when weight gained may not be lost completely. Women also tend to increase their body weight until their mid-sixties. Peak weight among men is up to the age of 50 to 55. Although both genders may lose weight in old age, it is thought that weight gain throughout middle age is simply a reflection of reduced activity.

Today, our normal diet tends to include foods that are manufactured, designed and marketed to be tasty and convenient. We can pop along to the local supermarket and buy ready-made meals that are quick and easy to prepare – with an exotic range of tastes. Alternatively, we can make a quick call and order a take-away. We also have fast food outlets where a hamburger, pizza or doner kebab can be purchased and devoured in a matter of minutes. Everything, it seems, is designed to save time by eating on the run, but with little thought of waistlines or health consequences.

Food to be found in packets or cans is unlikely to be fresh or full of goodness and flavour – unless the manufacturer decided to put it there! And the food that we choose may also be influenced by subtle marketing in terms of television advertising, posters and supermarket promotions. If it looks scrumptious, tastes delicious and there's a special offer, why not? Food manufacturers, and even restaurants, provide us with food designed to stimulate our senses by appearance, smell, taste and texture. Food will include additives to enhance colour and flavour, not to mention shelf-life. It is highly likely that additional sugar and salt, in all its formats, will be included.

So what is the answer? It really is simple, although not necessarily easy to pursue if you have a family to look after with all their varied tastes, timing and requirements. You should be aiming for a balanced and healthy diet, as described in Chapter 4. This will combine fresh fruit and vegetables to give you plenty of vitamin and minerals; healthy fibre in terms of cereals and potatoes to give you good carbohydrates, calcium and iron; fresh meat and fish for protein and more vitamins and minerals; dairy products for protein, calcium and vitamins; and small amounts of fat and sugary foods for energy, essential fatty acids and fat-soluble vitamins.

If we get this balance right, and cook in a healthy way, then it is unlikely that we will put on any weight (and it may even be that we lose some). But, in real life, we may have more than our fair share of take-aways, ready-made meals, snacks, chocolate and all the things that take our fancy. And, of course, there's also the odd tipple or two – and why not, after a lifetime's work! There's not much point in living if you don't allow yourself a few of life's little pleasures.

Actually, there is a point. Obesity is now the major cause of many of the diseases that try to see us into an early grave. And I wrote this book with the sole intention of helping you to put this moment off for as long as possible! Excessive weight can be responsible for arthritis, back pain, depression, high blood pressure, high cholesterol, piles, shortness of breath, insomnia, snoring, tiredness and varicose veins. If that's not enough, then think about the more serious illnesses such as cancer, diabetes, heart disease, hiatus hernia, osteoarthritis, kidney disease and strokes. Studies confirm that health and good nutrition co-exist – and conversely, when one deteriorates so does the other!

Evolving a healthier diet

On a personal note, developing a healthier diet for my family happened by accident, when we lived in the South of France for a few years.

The warm weather persuaded us to eat more fruit, vegetables and salads, and when we ate out we discovered that the French tend to create their meals around meat (and sauces) and vegetables, aiming for a variety of tastes rather than volume.

Unlike the English pub meals we had been used to, there was a marked lack of pastry and any potatoes that did find their way on to our plates were presented in a wonderful variety of guises – apart from the *pommes frites*!

Our favourite restaurant dishes were transferred to our French kitchen at home and a healthier diet gradually evolved without us even thinking about it.

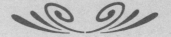

Of course, many people start to lose weight as they get older. There is a progressive loss of lean tissue throughout our lives, depending on our lifestyle, and an average of 40 per cent of our peak tissue may be lost by the age of 70 years. This results in a reduction in basal metabolic rate or BMR (see page 105) and consequently a reduction in our energy requirement. The loss of lean tissue, accompanied by weight loss, can also cause weakness and may discourage an elderly person from physical activity, leading to a spiralling situation of increasing inactivity.

There is much compelling evidence to suggest that diet, exercise and lifestyle play an important part in reducing the effects of ageing and the prevention of many diseases.

When it comes to healthy eating, we can learn a great deal from our neighbours, the French. Despite their well-acknowledged interest in – or even obsession with – eating, the French have a far better record when it comes to heart disease and other obesity-related health problems. I am not stating for one moment that all French cuisine is healthy, but they do make use of many more fresh ingredients than we do – have you ever noticed how many small food shops there are on the high street of even the smallest French town?

There is no doubt that a healthy diet will contribute to a healthier lifestyle, increasing your well-being and longevity. I have covered the area of diet in Chapter 4, so if you need to refresh your memory, go back and re-read this before we move on to talking about how to actually get rid of excess weight.

Are you overweight?

How do you know if you need to lose weight in the first place? Put another way, how much should you weigh? Most doctors use a simple measure called the Body Mass Index (BMI) to check whether you are overweight or not. Your BMI is your weight in kilograms divided by your height in metres squared. (You can also use imperial measurements – pounds and inches – but you must multiply the answer by 705 for the BMI reading.) If the result is 25 or more, you are classed as overweight. If it's over 30, you are clinically obese. And if it's nearer 35, that means you are severely obese and should have an **immediate** chat with your doctor. The table below shows how much you should weigh according to your height.

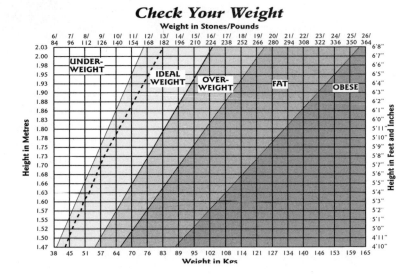

Check Your Weight

The important thing is to be within the limits of ideal weight. Obviously bone structure and body shape will vary from person to person and this will have a bearing on whether you are actually overweight or not. Your waist size can be a good guide – see the box below.

Obesity can also be assessed by measuring the percentage of fat in a person's body – the Body Fat Percentage. The ideal percentage of fat for a woman is between 20 and 30 per cent, and a man's around 20 per cent or less. Your Body Fat Percentage can really only be worked out by an expert, using skin-fold callipers, or electronic weighing equipment. You can buy electronic scales that will measure not only your weight but also your body fat percentage at the same time. They do this by passing a small (and entirely painless) electrical current through the body. The current measures any fat resistance (or bioelectrical impedance, as it's called) and calculates this against your height and weight, which are pre-set into the scales memory.

Check your waist size

Your waist size offers a fairly simple guide for diagnosis. The following table is based on recommendations by the Royal College of Physicians.

	Waist measurements		
	Ideal	**Worrying**	**Health risk**
Women	32 in/81 cm or less	32–35 in/81–89 cm	35 in/89 cm or more
Men	37/94 cm in or less	37–40 in/94–102 cm	40 in/102 cm or more

Weight check and progress

If you realise that you are overweight, then you need to work out how much you want to lose and over what period of time. Ideally, any weight loss should be gradual and evolve over months, rather than weeks. Crash and fad diets can be unhealthy and you are quite likely to end up putting more weight on than when you originally started! A good, healthy balanced diet, low in fat and sugar, coupled with some regular exercise, should see you shedding a pound or two every week, subject to your starting point. Sensibly you should consider a minimum of six months to lose weight progressively, perhaps even a year. If you are prepared to stick with it, you can achieve amazing results – a weight loss of just 1 lb a week would, over a year, add up to over **three and a half stone!**

So planning ahead is important to losing weight, and so is doing it at a slow, sustained pace. This way it will stay off. And because you are looking for long-term weight loss, don't worry about weighing yourself on a daily basis. Once a week, or even once a month, is fine. For the most accurate results, make sure that you do it at the same time, in the same place and on the same bathroom scales. Weight variations can occur when scales are placed on a carpet or bath mat, so always position the scales on a hard and level surface. Weigh yourself in the morning, without clothes, after going to the loo, and before drinking or having any breakfast.

Don't be obsessive about losing weight – muscle and body toning are just as important, even more so the older we get. Remember too that muscle is heavier than fat so if you are following an exercise programme, turning fat into muscle as well as dieting, you will not necessarily see much rapid weight loss. You will lose weight but, more important, you will be fitter and feel healthier. A body fat monitor will help to confirm this difference.

Monitor yourself

To give yourself some encouragement as you move towards your goal, get someone to take a couple of photographs of you on the first day of your new diet programme. The photographs should show you, ideally in a swimming costume or tight-fitting top and trousers, standing in a relaxed way, viewed from the front and from the side. With any luck, this should show all the features you're hoping to improve and as your figure tightens up, the difference you can see should encourage you to keep going. At the same time, start a diet diary (see page 48) in which you list everything you eat and drink during the day – and don't cheat – we can all easily kid ourselves! If your weight-loss programme doesn't bring results, the diary will soon show you if you have cut too many corners.

Get motivated

If you have an ambitious goal to achieve in the short term – say, a weight loss of one or two stones to get you into that special dress or swimming costume – resolve and determination to lose weight are vital for success. To test your motivation, ask yourself the following questions. Is losing this weight really important to you? Are you really prepared to make the effort? And are you willing to spend 30 minutes a day towards getting fit? You'll have to answer 'yes' to all of these questions before you move on. More than that, you have to mean it – if you aren't really determined to lose weight, you won't.

Is this a good time?

This may sound odd, but timing is important when it comes to trying to lose weight. If you are just about to give up smoking or you're facing a stressful situation such as divorce, bereavement or unemployment, then now may not be the time to think about changing your eating habits.

Choosing your diet

So you have now decided to lose some weight and want to choose a diet to achieve weight loss. Before embarking on any diet regime, bear in mind that a few minor eating adjustments (such as cutting down on snacking) and a little more physical activity (30 minutes' walking every day) could be all you need to do the trick – if you give it time. Alternatively, you might just need to make a few adjustments to your eating habits. As a general guide, men should eat no more than around 1,500 calories a day, and women should eat a maximum of 1,200. See Chapter 4 for plenty of advice on healthy eating. If you try to eat fewer sugar- and fat-orientated foods, combined with a little more activity, you may not even need to think about the word 'diet', which we tend to associate with 'deprivation'.

But if you feel that you really do need a proper, recognised diet, then you should think carefully about which type you go for. There are many diets available and I know many people who have tried them all. The thing to remember is that you are far more likely to succeed if you can find one that suits you – and your motivation. The more comfortable you are with it, the less likely you are to cheat, and by far the largest problem, when embarking on a new diet, is our tendency to kid ourselves. This is why a food diary can be such an important tool.

On the next pages I have listed the popular diets. Some may be better than others, but rather than just list those I rate highly I have included them all. It is worth knowing how they work so that you can make your own decision on which you think will be effective for you.

Note that the manufacturers of some diet products suggest that as soon as you reach your desired weight you can eat 'normally' again. However, you are likely to find that the weight rapidly returns unless you stick to a more healthy diet without any sugary snacks and sweets. In short, it seems to be that you have either to diet all your life, or to change to a healthy way of eating, which would be my preferred course of action.

High-protein diets

The most famous of these is the Atkins Diet, the first of the current range of high-protein, low-carbohydrate, high-fat diets. Its creator, Robert Atkins, maintains that this sort of diet ensures that fat is burnt quickly, thus decreasing obesity. Atkins also claims that by eating a low-carbohydrate diet, the body develops a mild form of ketosis, a condition that reduces the appetite.

It must be pointed out that Atkins's philosophy is in direct contravention of recommendations from the World Health Organisation and many other diet-related organisations around the world. Severe ketosis (which is actually usually linked with excessively low food intake or starvation) can be dangerous, causing mental confusion or even a coma in its extreme state. For what it's worth, however, I've known many people who have tried high-protein, lower-carbohydrate diets very successfully. If you do choose this type of diet, it is important to eat plenty of vegetables along with the protein, and to take vitamin and mineral supplements. (See Further Reading, page 201.)

The Hay Diet

The Hay Diet was originally devised by Dr William Hay in the 1900s. It was based on the belief that some groups of foods 'fight' each other, causing digestive problems. By avoiding eating such groups together, we simplify our digestion and detoxify our system at the same time. The philosophy is very simple but quite fussy to follow. For example, you must not eat proteins and carbohydrates in the same meal. This is because starches are broken down by alkaline saliva and proteins require gastric acid. Dr Hay also recommended that only wholemeal carbohydrates should be eaten rather than refined types – like white bread, white pasta, white rice, sugar, etc. Whether you believe the philosophy or not, this is good advice, and the diet undoubtedly works. But it may be difficult to comply with, especially when feeding other members of the family. For books on the Hay Diet, see page 201.

The Montignac Diet

This plan, originally devised by Michel Montignac, was written for business people in France, but ended up translated for the rest of the world (see page 201). Montignac's philosophy is not to mix proteins with carbohydrates (like the Hay Diet). He also divided his diet plan into two phases: during phase 1, the weight-loss phase, vegetables and salad are recommended with protein foods, with less emphasis on carbohydrates. In phase 2, the weight-maintenance phase of his diet, carbohydrates such as wholemeal bread, brown pasta and brown rice are allowed with sauces, but preferably not on the same plate as protein. Alcohol is allowed but measured carefully.

The Blood-group Diet

The idea for this one is that if you eat according to your blood type you will lose weight, build up your immune system and increase your energy levels. The idea was put forward in a worldwide best-selling book by Peter D'Adamo (see page 201). Adamo claims his diet will help to ward off diseases and deterioration in old age. His basic philosophy is based on an analysis of your body chemistry and how it absorbs vitamins and minerals.

High-fibre diets

The most famous of these is the F-Plan diet (see Further Reading, page 201). The theory behind it is a high intake of dietary fibre – potatoes, wholegrains, pulses, fruit and vegetables – up to double the amount you would normally eat. The bulk of what you take in fills you up but you end up consuming far fewer calories. High-fibre diets have a reputation for being healthy and reducing bowel cancer. Most high-fibre foods have a low glycaemic index figure (see page 65), which is recommended for any diet aimed at losing weight.

Meal replacement diets

The idea is that you swap one or two meals a day with a special meal replacement, which is calorie-counted and has all the essential nutrients included. These may be shake-type drinks, or soups or bars. Usually some fruit is allowed between meals. Because these diets are simple to follow they are very popular although they are boring. Weight loss will be fairly quick, especially if two meals are replaced, but you should beware of an equally fast weight gain after you stop.

Glycaemic index diets

Glycaemic index diets were originally devised for diabetics but are now marketed in various formats for slimmers. The glycaemic index measures the rate at which the blood-sugar (glucose) level rises when a particular food is eaten. The higher the rating, the more quickly it is absorbed into the bloodstream. For ordinary dieting purposes, you just need to know that the lower the GI, the lower the calorie content. See also Further Reading, page 201.

Low-fat diets

Low-fat diets obviously aim to reduce the amount of fat you eat, especially saturated fat (see page 50). The theory is that fat is full of 'heavy' calories and that the complex carbohydrates and proteins are low in calories, so if you reduce your fat intake and eat more protein and carbohydrate, you lose weight. The World Health Organisation recommends a low-fat, high-carbohydrate diet rather than calorie-counting as a way to avoid heart disease and obesity and for a healthy weight maintenance programme. However, unless you reduce your fat intake drastically, it may not work as a means to weight-reduction, and it can be dangerous to your health if you cut out all fat.

The Mediterranean Diet

The diet is simple – plenty of vegetables, salad and fruit, fish, shellfish, bread, pasta, and small amounts of meat or poultry. And, of course, virgin olive oil with everything. Both red and white wine are featured, but no potatoes or beer! If this sounds familiar, it is probably the type of food that you eat when you are on holiday – hence the name – and I can attest to its success as a weight-reducing diet.

The Rotation Diet

This diet was devised by Martin Katahn (see page 201). The number of calories you are allowed each day is regulated, starting with a very low number and increasing until you reach a fixed maximum, at which time you start again. Women are allowed 600 calories for the first three days, then 900 calories for another few days, then a week on 1,200 calories, followed by a week back on 600 or 900. Then you go back to eating normally for another week, before returning to the diet. It's the same for men except the calorie allowances are higher. The diet is obviously built around a low fat intake and reduced portions and daily exercise is recommended to help burn off calories.

The Zone Diet

This diet was developed by Barry Sears (see Further Reading, page 201) and advocates a diet that contains precisely 40 per cent carbohydrates, 30 per cent protein and 30 per cent fat. Sears claims that this perfect combination will produce optimum fat-burning and consequential weight loss, as well as reducing the incidence of heart disease and cancer. The favoured carbohydrates are those found in fruit and vegetables and no starches (potatoes, pasta, rice, bread, sugar, etc.) are allowed, except for oatmeal. The diet is very low in calories. It is also very fussy, although helpful recipes are given. It is arguable whether you lose weight because you are in the 'zone', or simply because of the reduced calorie intake.

Pills and supplements

Slimming pills and slimming supplements are available over the counter from chemists and health shops, by mail order and through the internet. They work in different ways: some products claim to 'block' calories or to bind to fat so that it is excreted before it is absorbed into the system. Some are diuretics and others are appetite suppressants. All claim minor miracles. I won't spend any more time on this, except to say, **don't bother**. They are, without exception, a waste of money and not the healthy route for longevity. Some are downright dangerous. You have been warned.

Weight management consultants

Weight management consultants will create a personalised diet for each client, based on their lifestyle. You will be asked to fill in and submit a detailed questionnaire, and experts will compile a list of recommendations, with a view to losing 1–3 lb a week over an initial period, with feedback as you progress. The aim is to make gradual adjustments, including exercise, to bring about a permanent healthier lifestyle. The service is offered by post or internet to keep consultancy costs to a minimum. If you find it difficult to keep to a diet on your own, this could be the answer. See page 202 for details.

Slimming clubs

Slimming clubs offer you a regime based on calorie-counting, although this may be expressed as an easy-to-follow points system for all foods. Using the system, you can eat whatever you want (within reason) up to a given number of points. The programmes usually last for around ten weeks and the weekly classes – which you must attend – help to maintain enthusiasm and commitment as well as providing a social element. Obviously, you pay for the course but you will receive plenty of information, recipes and support throughout. They will encourage you to eat healthily for life and persuade you to incorporate some regular and enjoyable exercise – ideal for those wanting to share their diet experiences every week or would like some company. See the listings in your local telephone directory.

Low-calorie diets

These plans work because you eat fewer calories than you expend in activity. This is a sure-fire recipe for success, but to stay interested you must choose a plan to suit your lifestyle. Some people prefer a diet that tells you exactly what to eat, others one with more flexibility. Low-calorie plans should also be low in fat, provide a wide range of foods and include lots of fruit and vegetables. Avoid those that involve eating a lot of one particular food and be sceptical of those that make claims to spot-reduce areas of the body. (This is virtually impossible – you can tone up individual areas by exercise, but you can't actually change the body shape you were born with.) As a general guide, women will lose weight on a daily calorie intake of 1,000–1,500 calories and men on 1,500–2,000 calories.

Slimming foods

The theory is that you eat slimming or 'healthy eating' foods in place of 'normal', higher-calorie foods. There's no doubt that the occasional slimmers' meal can be useful when time is limited, but relying too heavily on these foods does nothing to help people change to a healthier lifestyle, and low-calorie meals may be high in 'taste' additives, such as salt. Also, studies show that casual users of low-fat and low-sugar products do not reduce their calorie intake overall and may even think they can eat more of them! Slimming foods and meals can certainly help as part of a calorie-controlled diet, but you could probably create something tastier and with just as few calories with fresh ingredients at home.

Detoxification diets

Detox diets are basically very low-calorie diets that you follow for no more than a few days at a time. Fruit, vegetables and water are usually the only items eaten or drunk, with the idea being to 'rest' the digestive system, and flush out toxins. Some detox diets also suggest the use of cleansing herbs. Orthodox medical practitioners say that the body is perfectly capable of cleansing itself, and doesn't need this treatment to spring-clean it. There is also concern that people can feel weak and light-headed while on the diet – probably due to hunger. Detox diets don't have much scientific basis, but if you are in good health they should not do any harm. However, any weight you lose is likely to be regained as soon as you start eating normally again.

CHAPTER 7

Keeping Fit

There is little doubt that as we move into our fifties and beyond, our lives tend to become more sedate, especially as we ease away from our career – perhaps working part-time or being fully retired. The downside is that reduced physical activity can increase the risk of many illnesses that are associated with getting older. Gradual weight increases can also lead to obesity, with more consequences of ill-health. The upside of staying reasonably active will not only bring health benefits, it will help sustain both a physical and mental life way into old age.

But please don't panic. Keeping fit doesn't have to be about pumping iron, pounding the streets, or punishing yourself with sweaty gym workouts. It is simply creating a difference between a sedentary lifestyle and an active one, and one person's enjoyable fitness activity or exercise regime may be another person's nightmare! You are the only one who really knows whether you need to exercise a little more than you do at the moment. The odds say you do.

So where do you start? Certainly it's worth reading Chapter 8 to get an overview on both your existing health and fitness before starting any type of new activity or fitness campaign. If you are aged between 40 and 60 years old you should really have a health screening or medical check-up that includes a resting electrocardiogram (ECG) and, perhaps, an exercise stress test. The latter cardiovascular check is carried out while gently exercising on a stationary cycle or treadmill. Have a chat with your doctor, too.

As well as the health benefits, keeping active will make you look and feel better and give you more vitality.

Health checks

A health check will give you an idea of your current health and will be helpful in assessing what level of fitness you need to aim for. If you are undergoing any form of medical treatment you should check with the doctor, consultant or clinic that it is okay to start some new exercise regime. I am sure, in most cases, there will be no problem.

Although this chapter will encourage you to take up some physical activity, please consider that when you start any exercise for the first time, no matter how gentle, you will be adding a new stress to your body, which it isn't used to. So be especially careful if you have been inactive for a long period, or if you smoke or drink a lot. Always check with your doctor if you have a history of heart disease in your family, or suffer from hypertension or high blood pressure, or are very overweight.

Increased fitness can help all these conditions but increasing fitness levels will have to be gradual and carefully monitored. The less fit you are, the harder exercising for the first time will be, and if you are carrying a lot of excess weight, the challenge can seem a little daunting. In these circumstances it is worth first losing a little weight through diet as part of your fitness ambitions (see Chapters 4 and 6 – A Healthy Diet and Slim and Trim).

There are different forms of exercise, methods and fitness routines to suit everyone. And if you are particularly unfit, one special benefit is that you will see results very quickly, as the rate of improvement heads upwards very rapidly to begin with. Being able to reach a reasonable level of fitness involves two types of exercises: aerobic to improve cardiovascular fitness and anaerobic to build strength.

How fit are you?

So do you get breathless when you move at anything above walking pace? Are you puffed out after climbing one flight of stairs? As a rough guide to your fitness level, you can give yourself a do-it-yourself test to measure the efficiency of your cardio-respiratory system, but please bear in mind that everyone will be slightly different.

First you need to see how quickly your heart rate returns to normal after exercise. To do this, take your resting pulse rate while you are sitting or lying down, ideally first thing in the morning. Find your pulse on your wrist or neck and count the number of beats in 15 seconds and then multiply by four to get your 'resting pulse rate' in beats per minute. Check your results against the table opposite. If your resting pulse rate is in the 'poor' range, it would be inadvisable to embark on any kind of exercise programme for the time being. Make sure that you see your doctor for a health check before going any further.

If, however, your resting heart rate is 'fair' to 'excellent', you can now try speeding up your heart rate by taking some exercise. You can do this by stepping on and off a low stool or the bottom stair for **three minutes**, trying to keep a steady pace – one step every couple of seconds (women should aim for around 24 steps per minute and men around 26 steps per minute). Your full weight should be transferred to the stool or stair with both feet (left foot on, right foot on, left foot off, right foot off, etc.). When you have finished, rest for 30 seconds, then take your pulse rate, again counting the number of beats for 15 seconds and multiplying this figure by four. This figure is your 'recovery pulse rate' figure, in beats per minute.

Now compare your results to the table below. You can see that in both cases, the lower the figure, the fitter you are. As you exercise regularly, both rates should drop. You may never get into the 'excellent' range, but any improvement is better than none.

Resting pulse rate Women	Poor	Fair	Good	Excellent
40–49	100+	80–98	74–78	72 or less
50+	104+	84–100	76–82	74 or less
Men				
40–49	90+	74–88	66–72	64 or less
50+	90+	76–88	68–74	66 or less
Recovery pulse rate Women	Poor	Fair	Good	Excellent
40–49	116+	96–114	90–94	88 or less
50+	118+	100–116	92–98	90 or less
Men				
40–49	106+	90–104	82–88	80 or less
50+	106+	92–104	84–90	82 or less

Okay, so you are now thinking that maybe it's a good idea to think about getting a little fitter than you currently are. This is by far the biggest step. Just the word 'exercise' can strike fear into the heart of many of us, especially when we have become seasoned couch potatoes. Let's face it, we all know that taking regular exercise is a good idea, but that doesn't make it any easier to get started. So we'll take it slowly, one step at a time. Monitor your progress so that you can pat yourself on the back when you see or feel the difference, and keep reminding yourself of how well you are doing.

It is absolutely vital to choose an activity, exercise or fitness regime that you find easy and enjoyable at the start, so that you don't get bored quickly. If, for example, you try going to a gym and it just doesn't suit you, then look for alternate ways of exercising – like dancing, walking, aerobics, swimming, yoga, golf, tennis, etc.

Most of us abused our bodies in our thirties and forties – this is the age when we are more likely to be juggling stressful careers, children and household problems. It is also the time when many of us stopped taking exercise – usually because there just wasn't time – and now it's very difficult to get started again. But if you look at the panel on page 106, you don't have to be a scientist to realise that just a small amount of effort will improve your health and quality of life, regardless of your age or athletic ability.

When starting to exercise again after a long break, be honest with yourself, and don't overdo things. If you feel dizzy or sick, stop immediately and sit or lie down until you feel better. If you strain a muscle, let it heal before exercising again. There is no need to make yourself suffer, so forget the 'No pain, no gain' idea – it just isn't necessary. Provided you are in good general health, your common sense will tell you how much to do – but always speak to a qualified instructor when visiting a gym or keep-fit class.

Speaking of gyms, they can be quite expensive, but even if you are on a tight budget, you can still get active. You don't have to join some glamorous club – in fact, the only equipment you may need to invest in is a good pair of trainers or walking shoes. These are essential, however, as they will protect your back, knees, legs and feet, making any form of exercising more comfortable.

Now let's take a look at some of the different activities you can enjoy.

Walking

The idea that we can 'walk' for health and fitness may seem a little tame. After all, we have been walking all our lives. But national health studies show that most of us just have not been walking anywhere near enough. Due to the increase of gadgetry in our modern lives we work – and walk – less and less. We use cars, taxis, trains and buses more and more. Also escalators, lifts, electric doors, remote controls, television and internet shopping, home deliveries ... the list goes on and on.

Walking is probably the ideal low-impact, low-risk and low-cost activity. It is well documented that walking can have massive health benefits. Even walking at a moderate pace for as little as 30 minutes a day can significantly improve your cardiovascular system. Your heart will become stronger, your lungs more efficient and blood pressure can normalise. Walking can also improve cholesterol profiles, therefore helping to prevent coronary heart disease. Note that I did say 'moderate pace' – ambling along will do nothing at all for you! Walk as though you were a little late for a bus – you don't want to run, but you have to hurry ... and that should be about right.

Medical professionals advocate weight-bearing exercise as one of the best methods to keep our bones thick and strong. 'Weight-bearing' in this instance doesn't mean actually carrying any weight – the weight of your body is quite enough to make your legs work hard, so walking is extremely beneficial and has the added advantage of having a relatively low risk of causing injuries. Used in conjunction with a sensible eating plan, walking can also be very effective in helping weight management and weight reduction. However, health is not simply confined to our physical state. It also extends to our mental well-being. Many studies have been carried out that have shown walking to have a very positive effect on stress management and can help to increase the 'feel-good factor'.

There is nothing quite like exercising in the fresh air to leave you feeling totally invigorated. If you feel vulnerable walking alone, you could consider joining a walking club. Many clubs are aimed specifically at people in certain age ranges so you can look for one that suits you. Alternatively, you could organise one or two friends to join you on regular walks every week – as well as company, this provides an incentive to keep going, since you won't want to let each other down. Perhaps you could also investigate organised historic or scenic walks because, as well as offering good exercise, they incorporate points of interest, as well as stops at pubs or cafes for rest breaks. Your local council or tourist office should have some further information.

Another walking option is to leave the car at home more often and simply walk to the shops, work or a place of interest in your local area. Get into the habit of using the stairs instead of a lift or escalator. If you take a bus to work or go shopping, get off a stop or two earlier so that you have to walk further, and then do the same going home. You can start with short distances and gradually build up to longer walks. But make sure that you are wearing comfortable shoes. Start by walking at least one mile a day (it should take you 15–20 minutes) and gradually build up.

Ideally, begin your walk with a gentle warm-up of all the major joints in your body, including the spine. Take your joints slowly through their full, natural range of movement. This helps to lubricate the joints, reducing the risk of injury and increasing the comfort of the walk. Once this has been done, you should stretch all the main muscles of your body, particularly your upper and lower legs. You could also stretch the upper back and chest to prepare for the arm-swinging action. Use walls or fences for support. As an alternative to warm-up exercises, you can simply use a slow pace to start off, to warm up your muscles before walking briskly.

Now you are ready for the real walk. Your route should be planned carefully so you are aware of the type of terrain you will be walking on. You can choose known inclines or speed to alter the intensity of your workout. Preparation is also important as far as safety is concerned – see the panel below.

One of the great advantages of walking is that it can be done alone and at any time. However, if you prefer to walk with other people, you may like to join a walking group. They are extremely sociable and offer the added benefit of being slightly more structured in terms of intensity. A good coach can always structure a walking group so that every individual, no matter how fit they are, gets a workout. Contact your local gyms and health centres to see if there is a walking class near you.

Walking levels

You can start off walking at a comfortable and steady pace. It is important to focus on your posture, ensuring that you are standing up tall with your chin up, elbows slightly bent, shoulders back and striding out in a relaxed manner,

Tips for walking alone

- Stick to familiar areas with plenty of activity.
- Let a friend or family member know your route and estimated walking time. If there is no one to tell, leave a note at home in a visible place.
- Vary your route – it avoids boredom, and stops you being predictable to others.
- Try to walk in daylight. If not, choose a well-lit route and wear reflective clothing.
- If you feel you are being followed, turn and walk the other way, keeping to the same side of the road if you are being followed by a vehicle.
- Walk in the middle of pavements, not near alleyways, buildings or parked cars.
- Never wear expensive jewellery or carry valuables.
- Radiate confidence and purpose.
- Carry identification.

swinging your arms in a relaxed fashion. A faster pace of walking, known as 'power walking', will help to increase your fitness level. For this, bend your elbows to almost a right angle and emphasise the back swing of your arm. Don't let your arms swing out – keep them moving close to your body to generate a piston-type action. Your feet should land heel first, then toe, and you should try to avoid too much rocking of the hips. You may wish to switch between these two levels – the comfortable walk to warm up and the power walk for more intensive exercise. As your fitness increases, you will be able to sustain longer periods of power walking. You may then want to start including more hills on your route.

You can easily combine the different levels of walking with changes in the terrain, to increase the effectiveness and enjoyment of your walk. Try not to increase the duration or intensity of your walk any more than approximately 10 per cent per week. The number of times you choose to walk a week is up to you, but again, build it up slowly.

Hiking

Hiking is another form of walking that will definitely improve your health and it is an excellent way of combining healthy exercise with enjoyment, visiting places off the beaten track. You will need to invest in more specialist clothing for all weathers, as well as padded socks and walking shoes. There are so many places in the UK that can only really be explored by hiking, and it easy to understand why so many people get hooked once they start. Subject to the type or length of walks you undertake, when you walk, try to go at a pace that increases your heart rate, making you slightly out of breath, and use your arms as well as your legs. It really can make all the difference – and the miles will pass very quickly.

Cycling

Now is the time to rescue your bicycle from under that old pile of junk in the shed! It may not look like much now but a good dust-down, a drop or two of oil, perhaps a new tyre and you could be ready to go. We are not talking cycle racing or mountain biking – these are fast-growing sports but not for the faint-hearted. But if you would rather stick to the road than the undergrowth (like me), try using your bicycle to cycle somewhere specific, perhaps to the shops or to a friend's house. They – and you – are bound to be impressed; but remember that you have to pedal home again! A bonus is that as you are not driving you can have a social drink at the same time. (Don't overdo it, though – believe it or not, if you are involved in an accident, you can be prosecuted for riding a bicycle while under the influence ...)

Competitive sports

If you are a competitive person you may get more fun out of playing a sport. It is easy to think that you are too old to take up new sports, but with some coaching to start off with and plenty of time to practise you can achieve a reasonable level very quickly, and it will also provide an opportunity for a new social life and new friends.

Golf

Golf is one of those sports that you can take up – and excel at – at any age, and the handicap system allows beginners to play against better players without any embarrassment.

So maybe you're a potential Nick Faldo or Laura Davies. Go along to your local driving range and whack a few balls up, then perhaps try a lesson or two from the local golf professional. They will be used to teaching people of all ages and abilities and will give you plenty of helpful tips on your technique. All the equipment can be hired and, you never know, you might get hooked for good.

There's nothing quite like a game of golf on a spring or autumn morning to fill your lungs with fresh air and to take in the beauty of the season around you. Some nice weekends and holidays can be featured around the sport, especially if both partners play.

Tennis

Tennis is a good social sport and a lot of fun even if you are a total beginner (although most of us have played at some time – even if it was years ago). If you have a partner, go together. If not, a chat with the local club coach or secretary will put you in touch with like-minded people and a few lessons before you play your first 'match' will build up your confidence. If you don't like the idea of individual lessons, you can join a class of beginners. As you improve, you can start to think about playing matches – doubles matches tend to be light-hearted and can be lots of fun, improving both your fitness and social life. And who knows what mixed doubles can lead to!

Bowls

Both outdoor and indoor bowls have traditionally been the realm of the older generation, but recently many more young people have started to enjoy the sport, so it no longer has the 'oldie' stigma. Realistically, bowls won't do much for your aerobic fitness, but it can certainly help to improve your co-ordination, is very relaxing and sociable. And you can always walk to the bowling centre.

Working out

There are two options when it comes to working out. You can either go to a gym or sports club or you can do it at home. There are advantages to both. Gyms and clubs help to motivate you and are the more sociable option. But if you've got a few rolls of flab to get rid of, you may prefer to start off in the privacy of your own home – which is, of course, much cheaper!

Home workouts

It is really easy to work out in your own home. Exercise equipment, keep-fit videos and even magazines and books offer programmes for all abilities in the comfort of your house. Videos are an excellent start as they show regimes to suit all kinds of age groups, with easy-to-follow instructions and the accompanying music helps you to keep going. Also some of the television channels feature regular workout routines (you can always record them and use them again). If it all seems too complicated at first, you can watch the recording a few times until you learn the routine and can run through without thinking, just using the music. Some videos come in sets, designed for beginners, intermediate and advanced, which provide a good incentive to work your way through the series.

Working out on the cheap

Fitness equipment can come in all shapes, sizes and prices but again, you don't have to spend lots of money. Cans of food make excellent dumbbells for exercises, and a length of old washing line will make a skipping rope. Even a shopping bag loaded with a bag of sugar can be used to tone and strengthen muscles (sit on a chair, attach the bag to your foot, and lift and lower to strengthen leg muscles).

You can also use the stairs for exercise – try stepping on and off the bottom step (see page 97) or climbing them quickly, using your arms to propel you upwards, then slowly descend before turning around and repeating the process. This is just as effective as spending ages on one of those infernal stepping machines at your local gym. Work out a regime every day to be comfortable and habit forming.

Even the dreaded housework can be energetic, so put on some lively music and clean with vigour. Hoovering, brushing and sweeping will all work the muscles of your arms and upper body. Just think, not only will it help you to become fitter but your home will be exceptionally clean. Also, save money by washing your car by hand – all that stretching, cleaning, rinsing and polishing will increase your heart rate and circulation.

Of course, if you like gardening, cutting the grass with a hand mower will work your legs and back and digging the flower beds will make your lungs work harder and exercise different muscles in your body. So there are no excuses.

Home gym equipment

The convenience of having your own gym in your home is a luxury that few of us can afford. But it is amazing what you can achieve with a little space and a few pieces of simple equipment. And if you work out at home, you won't have to pay health club fees or travel to a crowded gym – for me, never a very attractive prospect, especially on a winter evening.

Exercise equipment designed to improve aerobic or cardiovascular fitness is particularly beneficial for older people. Before you buy any equipment, it is important to consider what you want to achieve, how much you can afford to spend, and the space that you have available. (Our spare guest bedroom, which houses a sofa bed, is our fitness room for most weeks of the year, and the equipment is easily stored away when we have guests staying overnight.)

The next step is to decide whether you want to get aerobically fit (that is, improve your lung capacity and stamina), or build up your strength, or increase your flexibility – or all three. This will influence the kind of equipment you will need to buy. For example, if you want a machine that will give you a cardiovascular and aerobic workout but do not require any resistance training, then an exercise bike or treadmill will meet your needs. Alternatively, if you want to build up some strength as well as be aerobically fit, then you may want to purchase some weights or a piece of resistance equipment. For almost everyone, a worthwhile addition is an exercise mat, which can be used for many floor exercises to improve your strength and flexibility, even when following a video. A good mat will cushion the impact on your joints and will make any floor exercises far more comfortable.

(While on the subject of videos and comfort, a television and video will be a useful addition to a fitness room or gym so that you can listen to music or watch your favourite programmes. Anything to keep you motivated and interested has to be a good investment.)

Don't buy any exercise equipment without trying it first and do be sure that it will keep you motivated. When using a piece of fitness equipment for the first time always be sure that it is operating on the lowest resistance setting and only increase the difficulty level once your fitness has improved.

Checking your progress

There are various checks that you can make to monitor your progress and levels of fitness.

Basal metabolic rate   Your basal metabolic rate (BMR) is the amount of energy required to keep your body working normally. Even when your body is resting, calories are still being used just to keep you functioning. Exercise will raise the metabolic rate as your body begins to work harder, thus burning more calories. This is why regular exercise is an important part of any weight-loss programme as you need to use more calories than you take in to achieve sustained weight loss. If you simply reduce your intake of food in an attempt to lose weight, the resulting shortage of calories can trigger a drop in BMR and your body will then attempt to overcome any shortfall in calorie consumption by conserving energy. This can make you feel weak or lethargic – and you won't lose weight very fast either!

Heart rate   Measuring your heart rate is important when working out on a regular basis. You need to make your heart work hard – but not too hard. It is positively dangerous to exercise above a certain level of heart rate, which is linked to your age. For maximum aerobic efficiency, you should aim to keep your heart rate within a safe target zone, which is around 70 per cent of your maximum heart rate. To work out your maximum heart rate, simply subtract your age from the figure of 220. So, for example, a woman or man of 50 will have a maximum heart rate of 170. A safe working zone would be 70 per cent of this figure, which is 119. Another method to check your workout intensity is to see how breathless you are when exercising. You should still be able to hold a conversation. If you can't talk because you are gasping for air, then you are certainly overdoing it.

A worthwhile piece of equipment is a pulse monitor, which you wear as a watch and is linked to your chest to detect your heartbeat. You can also measure your heart rate as described on page 96.

Working out at a club

There's a wealth of choice of sports clubs and leisure centres of all kinds. Check out your *Yellow Pages* to find out about your local facilities.

Health clubs and gyms

Ten years ago, a gym was likely to be small and privately owned, with little space and facilities, full of dedicated muscle fanatics or boxers. Nowadays, what was your local 'sweat shop' is now a health club, offering an extensive selection of workout machines, free weights, aerobics and yoga classes, often a swimming pool, serving drinks and healthy snacks in a luxury lounge or juice bar. There may also be a beauty salon or 'spa', offering a whole range of specialised pampering treatments to seduce you.

Reasons for getting more active ...

- Your heart will work more efficiently – during exercise the heart has to work harder to pump blood around the body, therefore it strengthens and increases in density.

- Your circulation will improve.

- Your lung capacity will increase as your lungs work harder and take in more air during exercise.

- Toxins built up in the body will be broken down and dispersed.

- Hormones (endorphins) released during exercise will leave you with a sense of well-being.

- Your metabolism will speed up, burning calories at a faster rate.

- Muscles will be toned, improving strength.

- Bone density will be increased with weight-bearing exercises.

- Muscles will be kept supple, improving mobility.

- Exercise can guard against serious illness, especially heart disease.

- Tension and stress, both mental and physical, will be reduced.

- Your energy levels will be greater.

- Feeling healthy will give you a more positive outlook on life in general.

But health clubs or gyms can still be frustrating places if you don't get what you pay for. For instance, if you join to use the gym and find that it is permanently packed with people on all the machines during your particular training times, you'll soon become disillusioned. Unfriendly staff can also be a problem – they should welcome you with a smile, not a sigh of boredom.

When you join, you should be invited for an induction session, where a fitness expert will assess your requirements and give you a programme to follow. It is then up to you to attend regularly to get the benefits. In many cases the novelty can soon wear off when there's a queue for popular machines, or it's difficult to get going after a hard day's work. If you have paid an annual subscription, you do not want to be wasting your money.

The best way to stay motivated is to find an exercise partner, then you can encourage each other. Then if you suddenly feel lazy or want to give the gym a miss, you'll be letting them down. It makes exercising a social event, too,

Checking out a gym or fitness centre

- Check out the staff attitudes. Are the receptionists friendly when you first go there? Are the gym staff well-informed, courteous and helpful? It is important to be surrounded by people prepared to encourage and support and motivate you.

- Ask to see the changing rooms. Are they clean and spacious? Are there plenty of lockers? Will you be able to enjoy a relaxing shower after your workout?

- Visit the gym too, preferably at a time when you would want to work out so that the atmosphere will be typical and you'll see what to expect. Are the machines all crammed in so that you can virtually touch the person on the machine next to you, or is there some space to breathe? Are there queues for some machines? Is the atmosphere hot and sweaty or pleasantly airy?

- If you do decide to join up, have a close look at the payment terms. Many health clubs will try to tie you in to annual agreements and may expect a hefty, non-refundable 'joining fee' in advance. Unless you're totally sure about your fitness commitment, it may not suit – and you could end up considerably out of pocket, so try to give yourself a 'get out' option if you need one. If you want to join for just three or six months as a trial, are they prepared to let you? If you get injured or have to work away from home, will the club be prepared to freeze or cancel your membership for a period?

perhaps with a drink afterwards. Also make sure you vary your programme at the gym and build enough time into your day so that exercise is not a last-minute rush or hassle. Set yourself goals relating to fitness or weight loss and body tone. Monitor your progress and reward yourself with special treats when you see or feel the difference. Keep reminding yourself of the fitness benefits.

Sports centres
A cheaper option than the full-blown fitness club is your local sports or leisure centre. Most of them cater for all ages, abilities and preferences, they offer a wide variety of activities in the same location, membership rates are much more reasonable than private clubs and there are always qualified staff on hand to make sure you carry out your chosen activity safely. Exercising with others is a great incentive and it is an excellent way of meeting people and making new friends.

Swimming

Water sports are a gentle way of introducing your body to more exercise – the water supports your weight and is therefore less stressful on joints and muscles. If you have never swum before, now is a good time to learn. It uses most of the main muscle groups, so it is one of the best sports for all-round fitness. If you find swimming a bit boring, you can try aqua-aerobics – exercise classes in the pool. As you would expect, movements are slow, but because the water provides resistance, you actually work harder than you realise. Aqua-aerobics is a great way to get fit without having to feel too energetic, especially if you can jump into a jacuzzi afterwards for a relaxing spa!

Swimming regularly is one of the best ways to get fit and stay fit. It suits all age groups and provides an all-round workout, improving the condition of your heart and lungs and working both your upper and lower body muscles. A hat may be useful if you have long hair, and goggles and a nose clip if the water is chlorinated. Most swimming pools offer lessons for improving techniques and fitness, and also set aside times and lanes for those who wish to swim in earnest.

Dancing

Enjoy a turn around the dance floor? Then why not take it up on a more regular basis? Even if your footwork isn't all that fancy, your local dance school should soon have you stepping in the right direction. Singles, couples and groups are all welcome and there are a variety of styles to choose from – ballroom, tap, modern, Latin American, line-dancing and rock 'n' roll. Dancing is an excellent, enjoyable form of exercise and very sociable at any age. American line-dancing is the latest craze – there's no partner required, it's a great exercise, and the cowboy hat is optional!

Stretching and relaxing exercises

So far I've talked a lot about vigorous exercise that involves exerting your body, making your heart and lungs work hard. But there are fitness regimes that require less effort, utilising various more gentle movements and stretches. These are particularly useful for someone with restricted flexibility, and can be particularly suitable for older people who are less mobile. Three of the better known stretch and exercise regimes are yoga, Pilates and t'ai chi. There are some excellent books and videos on all three, that you can use to get you started. See page 202 for addresses of contact organisations.

Yoga

Practised for thousands of years, yoga originally began as a philosophy to help concentrate the mind, and the postures were developed later to help with the meditation. Today there are various disciplines and styles usually consisting of gentle stretching exercises to release tension and harmful toxins from the body – perfect if you lead a stressful lifestyle. Usually yoga classes concentrate on suppleness, strength, stamina and concentration. If you are a beginner, it is wise to attend a yoga class with a qualified instructor who will teach the correct positions, but once mastered there is no reason why you can't practise yoga at home and at any time to suit you.

Yoga, through various postures, will help to strengthen muscles and improve flexibility. It can also help to alleviate back and neck pain, asthma, headaches, period pains and even aid digestion. Yoga maintains the full range of movement in your joints so it can help people with arthritis too. Most importantly, yoga will give you a feeling of health and mental well-being with its stress-busting exercises. Before starting, always inform the teacher of any medical conditions that you may have, or if you are recovering from an illness or injury.

Pilates

Developed by Joseph Pilates in the 1920s, this is a series of around 500 exercises using specially designed exercise equipment, although there are some exercise repertoires that can be carried out on a floor mat, so can be repeated at home after being taught. More complex than other forms of exercise, Pilates teaches breathing, body mechanics, balance, co-ordination, strength and flexibility. Its goals are similar to those of yoga, with both systems believing in individual progress in a non-competitive arena, with emphasis on stretching as well as the strengthening of the muscles.

From a fitness perspective Pilates will improve general fitness and improve posture. It is now used in sports training too, with tennis players, footballers and dancers using the system to improve their flexibility and strength. Pilates can also be used by any age group and often it is used therapeutically, to help with back problems, hips, knees, neck and joint injuries.

T'ai chi

The Chinese concept of fitness is a holistic, or 'whole body', approach. It doesn't rely on exertion and repetitive movements for effect, but attaches just as much importance to mental attitude as it does to strength and the flexibility of muscles and limbs. For those who are not robust, this is ideal as they can control their input to what is both comfortable and possible. Chinese medicine teaches that the body contains channels, called meridians, through which energy *(chi)* circulates. The meridians are thought to be linked to the major organs of the body, enabling the *chi* to flow freely between them, keeping them healthy. During illness, however, these channels become blocked, and an integral part of the treatment of disease is to free them. Exercise regimes such as t'ai chi are planned to promote the free flow of *chi* round the body. This means that it is performed in a relaxed manner, with the emphasis on slow breathing and a calm mind – an ideal approach for older people.

T'ai chi is, in fact, a martial art and requires years of long and rigid practice to become proficient in the fighting skills. It is this practice regime, consisting of a series of slow moves executed in a very relaxed way, that can actually build up stamina and strength, especially when performed as daily exercise. Because the exercise is gentle and controlled, there is very little chance of injury. T'ai chi classes can now be found in all parts of the country, but it is important that you choose an instructor who is properly qualified, and accredited to one of the recognised professional bodies.

Fitness clothing

Once you've decided on the type of exercise you want to do, you need to get yourself kitted out. The most important thing about taking exercise is to have fun, so it follows that what you wear needs to be comfortable and make you feel good. The sportswear industry is constantly updating the fabrics and styles they use to make exercise clothing more versatile. Super-absorbent materials have been developed that help to draw sweat away from your body, leaving you feeling dry and comfortable. Some keep you warm, some keep you cool, some cling and move with your body, and others are a looser fit for a more casual look. All you have to do is choose your outfit to suit your activity.

It's a good idea to think about 'layering' your clothing. Trapped air between each item helps to keep your body warm. Layering is also the most versatile way to dress, as you can strip off as you get hot and pile the clothes back on as you cool down. For the 'inside' layer, you have a choice of crop top, short- or long-sleeved T-shirt and shorts, or leggings. When you're warmed up or in the middle of your workout, these are what you should be wearing so that your body is able to sweat and disperse moisture without overheating. If you're training outside or just starting your exercise, you should wear another layer on top – a sweatshirt and jogging trousers, or the more modern kick flares – to warm your muscles ready for some intense activity. Finally a wind and water-resistant jacket and some protective trousers will keep the elements out if you intend to go for long walks or runs, or any outdoor activity.

Women should wear a good support bra or bra top suitable for exercise; there are plenty available. It needs to fit well and have good support under the breasts and over the shoulders. Don't be afraid to try one on and have a little jump around to see if it does the job!

Health farms

So far this chapter has been full of words like 'exercise', 'regime', 'practice', 'exertion' and 'workout' – it all sounds pretty energetic. But if you want to kick-start your fitness regime with a little pampering, you could give yourself an incentive and a treat at the same time by booking a break at a health farm or a hotel with leisure facilities. Enjoying some exercise along with plenty of pampering is the ultimate in luxury and can give you the incentive you need to embark on a healthier lifestyle.

If you've previously dismissed health farms as being either too expensive or elitist, it may be time to think again. Most of them are full of ordinary people who just need a few days away from the pressures of modern living. Prices can compare favourably with ordinary weekend breaks, and although the entry price may be slightly higher, once you are there, you don't usually have to spend much more, as meals and treatments are usually included.

Value for money

For a real break away from it all and the best value for money, a three-night stay is advisable, to give you time to unwind properly and really get the most from your stay. A three-night midweek stay will be cheaper than a weekend and many health farms now offer one-day visits, with prices depending on what you choose to do. If you stay for a week or longer, the price per day goes down, and most will do seasonal offers – usually during summer and just before Christmas – so it's worth checking out before you book. Sharing a room with a friend is also a cheaper option than going it alone, though you won't feel out of place if you do go on your own, as the atmosphere is usually very friendly.

Included in your basic price are accommodation, all meals and some drinks, use of the gym, pool and sauna, exercise classes and usually one treatment session. However, many now do special packages that include several treatments (e.g. a spa break, pampering break, toning break, etc.) in the price. Any extras will be added to your bill.

There are now dozens of health farms, spas and clinics dotted throughout the country, and many more abroad if you really want to escape. But before you make your choice, take a look at the range of treatments and facilities that are on offer and decide what your main priorities are: pampering and relaxing; sports and fitness; pools and saunas; healthy eating; or natural and complementary therapies.

Relaxation

While the whole experience of the health farm is designed to relax you and melt away stress, there are some treatments that are specifically designed to help you unwind.

Flotation This is designed to relax the body by losing all sense of gravity, sound and sight. You will either lie in a warm salt bath, floating on the water, or resting on a water-resistant sheet, which floats on top of the water (dry flotation).

Massage One of the best de-stressing and relaxing treatments available, massage comes in many guises. Aromatherapy massage, which uses essential oils, is a very popular method, as are shiatsu and massage using vibrating pads.

Stress-management classes Held at some of the health farms, these are designed to help you learn to avoid, as well as cope with, everyday stresses once you're back at home.

Water-based facilities

Almost every health farm or spa will have a swimming pool. Also available are saunas, Turkish baths and jacuzzis, which are wonderful ways to help you unwind. Health spas often specialise in water-based health treatments such as hydrotherapy baths to ease away aches and pains, jet streams and thalassotherapy, which offers treatments that use marine extracts such as algae and seaweed.

Complementary therapies

Some health farms specialise in complementary therapies, with the aim of addressing inner health and aiding relaxation, rather than pampering beauty treatments. If this is the kind of break you want, then you are best to book into one of these specialist health farms. Most centres, however, now offer a range of the more popular therapies such as aromatherapy, acupuncture, shiatsu and reflexology (see Chapter 10).

Pampering and beauty treatments

These are among the most popular treatments, so you may be advised to book them in advance. According to the health farms, the reason most people – men and women – give for visiting them is to relax and be pampered, and the beauty treatments are also very popular, with massages and facials being the most requested treatments.

Body treatments are numerous and can include mud packs, body wraps, plus detoxifying, exfoliating and anti-cellulite treatments. Hair removal treatments, such as waxing and electrolysis, are popular too.

There will be beauticians on hand to give make-up lessons and advice on skin care. Manicures and pedicures are a popular choice, and are also often included in the basic price. Some health farms have sunbeds, if you're hankering for a bit of winter sun, but be aware of the risks of over-exposure to damaging rays.

Fitness activities

If you want to make a start on getting fit, most health farms will do an assessment and devise a fitness plan for you. It is a good place to go if you want to try out a new sport or start an exercise routine and ideal for people who may be apprehensive about going to a gym for the first time.

Health farms are now equipped with a range of facilities, as well as qualified fitness instructors and personal trainers. For people wanting to explore a fitness regime, they can devise a personal exercise plan that you can continue with when you get home. Practically every health farm will have a gym, but it's worth checking out what type of equipment they have, especially if you are going specifically for the fitness, as some are better than others.

Aerobics and fitness classes are often included in the price and tend to be well attended. Many health spas will offer aqua-aerobics classes too. Some will have squash and tennis facilities, including qualified instructors, while others have golf courses with a professional on hand to offer some advice or give lessons. Even outdoor activities such as walking, hiking or cycling are usually catered for, as most health farms tend to be located in beautiful countryside.

Healthy eating

You can expect a good selection of healthy food, whichever health farm you decide to visit, though some are more adventurous than others. Meals are usually calorie counted, and there are plenty of fresh salads, vegetables and fruit to choose from. Some will serve wine with meals, but alcohol usually isn't encouraged. If you are trying to lose weight, then a nutritionist may be on hand to give you advice and suggest a diet.

The crash diet approach of losing pounds in a few days is now outdated, and health farms don't encourage it. Instead, they help you to take a longer term view of weight loss, combining it with exercise and a healthy diet, with less emphasis on losing weight and a greater interest in healthy eating.

CHAPTER 8

‿ଓ ৡ৲

Good Health

If you had just one wish, what would it be? Health, wealth or happiness? Apart from a win on the lottery, good health would come high on most people's wish list. It's something we all take for granted – until it's suddenly gone. Only then do we realise just how important it is.

Don't take your good health for granted – take care of it.

If you are healthy now, then you can probably remain so. But as we get older we have to be more aware of the sort of things that can go wrong. Getting old does not have to mean you are heading for illness or bad health. Many of the problems encountered when we get past 50 years of age are due to bad lifestyle habits, which can easily be recognised and consequently modified. In this book, I have covered many strategies to help slow down the ageing process. A healthy diet, regular exercise and an active mind can keep ageing at bay, while sensible use of natural remedies and therapies can help to prevent many of the ailments and unwelcome effects associated with it.

It is important to know how your body ages and what the warning signs of illness you should be looking out for. Your doctor could play a crucial role in your health, especially in later years, so now is the time to get on good terms with yours, as well as having regular check-ups and health screening. Identifying illnesses in the early stages will greatly increase the chances of successful treatment.

Regular screening

Ideally, people over the age of 50 should have a health check at least once a year, especially if a particular complaint needs to be kept under observation. Regular screening will also give you peace of mind. Some people can even worry themselves into an early grave by getting anxious about illnesses that they do not actually have! So the message is to be safe and sure, always remembering the old adage, 'Prevention is better than cure.'

If you go for a check-up, your doctor will usually monitor your blood pressure and cholesterol levels and test your urine. For women, a cervical smear may well be given, as well as a breast examination. Your doctor may take note of your height and weight to check your BMI (see page 86) or take a simple waist measurement to check for excessive weight. If you have particular concerns or have a family history relating to a specific illness such as cancer or heart disease, other tests may be carried out and possibly performed at another clinic or hospital. These tests could include a blood test, lung function, an electrocardiogram to monitor your heartbeat and a chest X-ray (especially important for smokers).

Screening procedure

I recently arranged for health screen checks for my wife and myself. We arranged to go to separate clinics so that we could compare notes afterwards.

Before booking our checks, we shopped around to see what was available. The most obvious route was to go through a well-known medical insurance company. Many insurance companies now offer individual screenings to anyone who requests one – there is no need to be a member or subscriber to their medical insurance cover. The first one I tried suggested their 'premier' health assessment, which is designed to help detect any early stages of heart disease, and included a dynamic cardio-respiratory exercise test examining heart, lungs and circulation. There were also tests on blood pressure, respiration, metabolism and fitness, and an ECG, plus general health tests to detect any problems relating to blood, urine, eyesight, hearing, nutrition and stress. All pretty comprehensive, but with a price tag to match – the whole thing came in at a shade under £500.

After some further research, I discovered an alternative screen testing facility for less than half the price, with a menu of optional extras to suit your requirements. This was through a national screening network, who arrange health screenings throughout country. Their costs are lower because they do not have dedicated clinics to maintain, utilising the facilities of doctors surgeries or clinics. You pay for the doctor's time and the laboratory fees, with minimal administrative overheads, which is ideal for people on a tight budget.

Their standard examination will study your personal and family medical history, take height, weight and other body measurements, perform a complete physical examination, including testing peak flow lung function, eyesight and hearing, urine analysis and monitoring blood pressure. Blood samples are also taken for analysis by a specialist laboratory, who carry out over 25 different tests, with a view to establishing accurate levels of cholesterol and other substances. These may show imbalances in the body long before any physical effects are apparent. An electrical tracing of heart activity is taken, analysed and interpreted by a consultant cardiologist, with feedback provided by the examiner.

The menu of extras includes chest X-rays, a prostate cancer test for men and a variety of tests specially for women, including self-check training in breast examination, a cervical smear and gynaecological examination. So you can choose a screen test to suit you, subject to your gender and requirements. You can also specify whether you want a female or male doctor, although this may restrict your choice of venue and may also mean you have to wait a little longer.

His health screen

You are offered a choice of venue for your screening – usually within a 20-mile radius of your home or place of work, subject to personal requirements. I chose to have my health screen in Chatham as I live in Kent. I had been given a form to fill in prior to my visit. The first part of the screening was a short talk with the doctor about the details covered in my form, including any previous medical history and any present concerns that I had. Then followed a thorough physical examination, checking heart, lungs, blood pressure, reflexes, etc., and the urine sample I had earlier provided was analysed on the spot for signs of diabetes or kidney infection. My weight and height were measured and then the doctor calculated my BMI reading and took blood samples for laboratory analysis (I opted to give an extra sample for a separate prostate test). He took my resting ECG (be warned: chest hair has to be shaved to accommodate the sensors) and the resulting graphs were sent to a consultant cardiologist for analysis.

The doctor discussed my weight and fitness levels, although he didn't actually discuss my diet. That said, there was no real need; my diet is very healthy, my fitness levels good and I keep a regular eye on my weight. I was in and out of the doctor's surgery in around one hour.

Her health screen

Since she frequently travels into London, my wife Sue had chosen a clinic based in London's Harley Street for her screening. Her examination took about an hour, with similar tests to mine. She had filled in a health questionnaire beforehand, and the doctor went through it with her, asking about her family's health history, her general daily diet and any health queries that she may have had.

Next came a physical examination where her joints, muscles, reflexes, moles, nails and tummy were examined. The doctor also listened to her chest and checked her spine for any abnormalities. She took Sue's blood pressure, and then wired her up for her resting ECG test, attaching pads to her chest area, ankles and wrists.

The doctor made a careful check of the breasts for any lumps or bumps, explaining along the way how Sue should check them regularly herself and the techniques involved (see page 133). Sue's sight and hearing were also checked, including a test for colour blindness. She was weighed and her height, chest, waist and hips were measured. During this period her urine sample (given before the screening) was read and analysed.

Results

After a health check like ours, you should receive a written report. Both of ours were received about two weeks later, with the doctor's notes on the examination and a detailed report on the results of all the tests on both blood samples and ECG. Even if, like us, you are given a clean bill of health, a health screen will still supply peace of mind – and, more importantly, will throw up anything particularly threatening perhaps before it would have been detected in the normal course of events.

Be aware

Many older people do not visit their doctor often enough. It is important to identify any problem early. Symptoms that persist for a more than week or so, or seem to be getting worse should always be checked. Always keep an eye on how you feel and don't be afraid to ask to see your doctor especially if you have any chest pains, or a cough that persists for weeks instead of days. Keep an eye on skin ulcers and cuts that don't seem to heal quickly. Check for any new lumps or bumps – women should examine their breasts regularly and men should do the same for their testicles. If you suddenly have irregular or unusual bowel motions, especially blood in the faeces, this should be investigated immediately. Women should be aware of any unusual vaginal discharge.

Cardiovascular health

The cardiovascular system involves both your heart and circulation. Blood moves around the body carrying all-important oxygen and nutrients to the body's cells. As we grow older, the cardiovascular system will become less efficient, moving more slowly and possibly less rhythmically. Exercise and control of your diet, particularly your intake of cholesterol (see Chapters 4 and 7) can help to improve cardiovascular performance. Cholesterol, although an important substance for the body, can be especially dangerous if present in high levels (see page 56). If your heartbeat is seriously irregular and interferes with your everyday life, it can normally be corrected with a pacemaker.

Research shows that some people are more at risk than others when it comes to heart disease. It is important to know your family history in terms of previous heart problems or conditions so that you can take any necessary preventative measures and perhaps adjust your lifestyle to allow for this. You should also make your doctor aware when you speak to him or her. Those in the category of high cardiovascular risk are smokers, people with high blood pressure and high blood cholesterol levels, people who are obese, those who do little physical activity and diabetics. Exercise is important as it increases the amount of oxygen transported to the heart. Always check with your doctor before exercising, especially if you already have a heart condition such as angina or high blood pressure. Start with gentle exercise like walking, and keep within a comfort zone – don't continue if you're breathless, tired or in pain.

Blood pressure

Blood pressure rises with age because our arteries naturally harden and narrow as we grow older. Blood pressure can also rise if we are under conditions of stress or high emotions. Excessively high blood pressure is dangerous because it can lead to other complications, such as kidney failure, strokes or heart disease. A check-up by your GP should detect any problems, which can often be effectively controlled through both diet and exercise, although drugs may be necessary. If you are diagnosed as having high blood pressure, you can help to reduce it immediately by making a few simple lifestyle changes. These include minimising stress, reducing your intake of salt and fat, cutting down on alcohol, losing excessive weight and stopping smoking.

Strokes

If the blood can't flow around the body properly, blood supply to the brain may be reduced, resulting in a stroke. Although strokes can be very dangerous and debilitating, many people still make a total recovery, but the chances of this are obviously subject to the severity of the stroke. The same diet and exercise measures to help protect your heart and cardiovascular system will also guard against strokes.

Respiratory health

By taking good care of your lungs you can improve their capacity and, more importantly, their resistance to disease. Problems with breathing can become more noticeable as we get older, as the body becomes less flexible and air volume in the lungs is reduced, making them less efficient. The lowered immunity of older people can also make simple respiratory illnesses more serious, leading to complications.

As always, continuing to stay fit in your later years is the best way of protecting yourself from lung disease. Regular exercise will increase the capacity of the lungs by increasing the elasticity of your body. People who sing or play a wind instrument have improved lung capacity, so taking either of these up as a hobby could prove beneficial for the lungs in the coming years ahead.

Even though you may never have suffered with asthma, it can develop later in life through age, illness or smoking. Asthma is an allergic respiratory condition, characterised by paroxysms that make breathing difficult. Attacks can be distressing but there are excellent drugs available that quickly relax the airways and give immediate relief. Should you have an attack, it is important to stay calm. Avoid taking shallow breaths and use your diaphragm to help you breathe. Asthma may be a chronic condition, or it may be triggered by an allergic response to something close to you. Common causes are dust, animal fur, smoky atmospheres and environmental pollution. I suffered with regular asthma attacks during my childhood and think the cause may have been the feathers and rubber glue that my mother used in her trade of making hats! Smoking in my youth didn't help matters either, but since quitting the weed and taking up regular sports activities, I have never looked back. Avoiding dairy products may help symptoms as these increase the amount of mucus manufactured by the body.

Severe colds, flu and coughs present a greater threat to our respiratory health as we become more elderly. Lung complaints can become dangerous if not taken seriously or treated straight away. Infections can take hold when the immune system is low and can lead to illnesses such as pneumonia, bronchitis and emphysema. Make sure that you see your doctor if infections do not clear up quickly. Influenza can be very serious, causing aching muscles, high temperatures, hypothermia and dehydration, and aggravating any existing respiratory conditions. If you have asthma or any other respiratory condition, you should speak to your doctor about having a regular flu injection every winter. It is also recommended that everyone over the age of 60 should have one.

A healthy digestive system

Throughout this book emphasis is placed on what we eat and how our diet can affect our health. The food we put into our mouths is important and so are the mechanics of dealing with it. It is important that we chew our food well and moisten it with saliva, before it is digested in the stomach and small intestine.

Ten common symptoms to watch out for

1 **Tiredness**   If you feel constantly tired without any apparent reason (and are still getting plenty of sleep) arrange to see your doctor.

2 **Weight loss**   Sudden weight loss without any dietary changes should always be investigated, just in case it is the first sign of illness.

3 **Cuts and bruises**   Cuts that don't heal quickly or severe bruises that appear with just a slight knock should be checked out.

4 **Difficulty in swallowing**   If you have difficulty in swallowing food or liquid, then let your doctor investigate.

5 **Rectal bleeding**   Although haemorrhoids remain the most commonest cause of rectal bleeding, please have any such signs checked by your doctor, just in case there may be a problem with the bowel.

6 **Change in bowel habits**   Any change in bowel habits lasting more than a couple of weeks should be reported to a doctor. This could be unexplained diarrhoea, constipation or unusual sensations in the bowel.

7 **Blood in urine**   This is most commonly caused by a urinary infection, but could be a sign of more serious bladder problems.

8 **Headaches**   Everyone gets headaches, but it is worth checking them out if painkillers have no effect, or they are associated with nausea, vomiting or blurred vision.

9 **Vaginal bleeding**   Unexpected bleeding after the menopause and bleeding after intercourse should be investigated by your doctor.

10 **Jaundice**   Any yellowness of the skin should be assessed. There can be many reasons but it's best to identify the problem quickly.

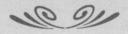

Once the nutrients have been absorbed and excess water removed, the waste is excreted. Each part of the digestive system needs to function properly to allow the body to absorb all the important nutrients it needs to protect the rest of our body, so problems with the digestive system can sometimes lead to other unrelated illnesses.

Eating a regular and healthy diet will help to maintain a healthy digestive system. Just avoiding caffeine products, such as tea, coffee and colas, and eating smaller portions of food can help to reduce heartburn, as can eating less fatty, acidic and spicy foods. Drinking plenty of fluids, ideally water, and exercising regularly can also help to relieve indigestion and heartburn. The mouth plays an important role in digestion – eating slowly and chewing well make it easier for the stomach to digest food. Decayed teeth or badly fitted dentures can help to create digestive problems, so be sure that all is well at the point where the process starts. A weight-loss tip is to chew your food at half the speed you normally do. This means that you will probably feel full before you complete your meal, and will be able to decline all those tempting second helpings or desserts on offer!

Anxiety itself can also trigger diarrhoea or stomach ache, and stress or worry can lead to people reaching for alcohol or comfort foods to hide the problem. This will play havoc with the digestive system, especially over a period of time.

Hiatus hernia

As we get older our body tissues become less pliable and can start to sag. The most common result of sagging tissues is a hiatus hernia, which happens when the stomach muscles weaken and part of the stomach protrudes up into the chest. It is reckoned that at least over half of people over the age of 60 have a hiatus hernia! Many have a mild version without any symptoms and it is never diagnosed. Usually it makes little difference to the digestive system, although it can sometimes lead to painful indigestion. Treatment can involve losing weight, eating little and often, and giving up smoking. Antacids can help to reduce any heartburn and avoiding bending or lying down after meals may give some relief. If symptoms are severe, surgery to repair the hiatus hernia can be undertaken. This is a major operation where the protruding stomach is pulled back into place and permanently secured.

Diverticular disease

Diverticular disease can occur when the support of the colon walls begin to sag, and small pockets form. Partly digested food can build up and then ferment in these pockets, causing painful bloating and stomach pains. Diverticulosis is very common in the Western world, but is virtually unheard-of in Eastern and African countries where the diet is largely made up of fibre, fruit and vegetables. Insoluble fibre (see page 51) is important in our diet to prevent diverticulosis, and will also promote regular bowel movements.

Healthy bones

Our bones – or skeletal system – provide a rigid structure for the muscles to work against and also support our internal organs. As we get older, our bones become less dense and more brittle. This makes people more prone to bone fractures as they get older. Also, with wear and tear, the cushioning in the joints is reduced and ligaments will shorten, leading to a loss of flexibility.

Osteoporosis

Bones are not solid: they are made up of a honeycomb of bone cells. As we get older, our bones become more porous. By our early thirties, our bones will have reached their maximum size and density and after that, bone density begins to decrease, at the rate of about one per cent a year. It is a natural process but it can have a detrimental effect on many people's lives. Osteoporosis, the bone-thinning disease, occurs when the holes in our bones become larger, making the whole structure thinner and weaker. This is particularly common in post-menopausal women because of the lack of oestrogen production (see page 129). Women who experience an early menopause, or stop menstruating because of excessive dieting or exercise, will have depressed levels of the hormone oestrogen – which helps our bone regenerate – and as a result will be at greater risk of osteoporosis. For this reason, many doctors now encourage menopausal women to take hormone replacement therapy (HRT), to reduce this risk (see page 125).

It is worrying that most people won't even know that they have this debilitating disease until a minor fall leads to a broken bone. By then, it can be in its advanced stages and can even prove fatal – it is estimated that 15,000 women

Osteoporosis prevention – dos and don'ts

- Eat a well-balanced diet with plenty of fruit and vegetables, as well as foods rich in naturally occurring oestrogen, such as soya products, linseed, green and yellow vegetables and gingseng, and calcium.

- Take regular weight-bearing exercise – at least three or four sessions each week. This helps to increase the uptake of calcium by bones. Try jogging, brisk walking, playing racket sports, lifting weights, low-impact aerobics, skipping and even squeezing tennis balls.

- Take a supplement containing calcium, fish oils and evening primrose oil to help maintain bone mass.

- Restrict your alcohol intake to no more than seven units per week and do not smoke – research has shown that women who stop smoking at the time of the menopause may reduce their hip fracture rate by as much as 40 per cent!

die each year following an osteoporotic hip fracture. However, it is possible to stop it getting this far. If you are concerned, or you know that osteoporosis runs in your family (there is a clear genetic factor), ask your doctor to arrange for you to have a bone density test. Blood tests may be done to check for calcium and bone chemistry, as well as for other diseases that have similar symptoms. Other diseases that can cause secondary osteoporosis, such as an overactive thyroid, can also be detected this way.

If you are given the all-clear, it's still wise to consider yourself at risk – and take positive steps to strengthen your bones. Whether you choose to tackle this yourself by changing your dietary and lifestyle habits, or use medical methods of treatment, it is never too late to start.

Calcium

Calcium is particularly important for maintaining strong healthy bones. However, many people consume less than the recommended daily intake of 800 mg and are at risk of reaching middle age with a low bone mass, making them more susceptible to osteoporosis. Because calcium is not easily absorbed, it's important to make sure you include lots in your diet. The best sources of calcium are milk, dairy products, green leafy vegetables, nuts, eggs, bony fish, orange juice and hard water. A daily supplement of calcium can also boost your intake, especially if it's combined with essential fatty acids (EFAs), which will aid absorption.

The reproductive system

As we grow older, our reproductive systems, like most of our bodily functions, work less efficiently, although men do rather better in this particular area – there are plenty of documented cases of men fathering children when in their seventies, or even later. For women, the situation is different. Women are programmed to reach their reproductive peak in their twenties, and for most women, their fifties marks the time when the ovaries cease to function and they can no longer have children.

The menopause

As I have said, the menopause usually occurs at around 50 years – the average range is actually 47 to 52 years of age. Premature menopause may occur in women who have had a hysterectomy, and smokers tend to enter the menopause two years earlier than average.

There are many views of how women should deal with the menopause. It is a natural event and shouldn't be treated as an illness (although in Western society we have tended to do this), but it is a very important time of a woman's life. Doctors may prescribe extra hormones (see Hormone replacement therapy, below) and many women may just try to make the best of what can be a very trying few years. But since it is widely acknowledged that diet and lifestyle play an important role in how the menopause affects women, it is possible to take a more positive attitude, by preparing for the menopause before it occurs.

The clearest sign of the onset of the menopause is the gradual reduction in the frequency of monthly periods. (It is worth noting, however, that the complete cessation of menstruation is the very last stage. This means that many women going through the menopause may still be very fertile – so beware!) There are many other signs and symptoms, most common being hot flushes, which can occur many times during the day and last from a few seconds up to 30 minutes. Some women turn red and sweat profusely, some have palpitations, others will just experience body heat. Hot flushes are frequently experienced during the night ('night sweats'). The walls of the vagina become thinner as the levels of oestrogen fall, and blood flow is restricted causing a lack of lubrication, leading to uncomfortable dryness and reducing libido (sex drive). Paradoxically, regular sexual activity stimulates the blood flow into this area and can help to reduce the dryness. Other symptoms of the menopause are dry skin, dry hair, weight gain, tiredness, weak bladder and aching limbs and joints. There may also be problems with psychological changes, due to the hormone imbalance, which can lead to lack of self-esteem, mood swings, depression, insomnia, forgetfulness and a loss of libido. Thankfully it is unusual for women to experience all of the symptoms.

Hormone replacement therapy (HRT)
Available in different forms such as patches, pills and implants, HRT is a means of providing the female sex hormone oestrogen, which the body stops producing naturally after the menopause. It is prescribed for a variety of reasons, one of the main ones being to prevent osteoporosis (see page 123). Oestrogen slows the loss of old bone and stimulates the continuing production of new bone. Studies have shown that even in women with established osteoporosis, HRT can slow further bone loss and reduce the risk of a fracture.

However, some women may experience unpleasant side-effects, which may prevent its use in the long term. Up to two-thirds of women come off HRT within the first year because they are unable or unwilling to tolerate it.

So should you take HRT? The answer is, there are pros and cons. There is no doubt that it reduces the incidence of osteoporosis and associated bone fractures, such as broken hips, which affect many older women. It also works for hot flushes, night sweats and vaginal dryness, and many women report that the condition of their skin and hair improves.

However, there are undoubtedly some disadvantages to HRT, with minor side-effects occurring in around 15 per cent of users. These include breast tenderness, weight gain, nausea, headaches, itchy skin, rashes and fluid retention. There is also an increased danger of blood clots. With some types of HRT monthly bleeding continues – or may indeed return after it has stopped – although some brands produce three-monthly bleeds and others none at all (the latter can usually only be taken if the periods have actually stopped of their own accord, however). There is also some data that suggests there may be an increased risk of breast cancer if HRT is taken for a longer period – five to ten years.

The natural alternative

Many women are put off the idea of HRT and prefer instead to advocate the natural way of dealing with the menopause. If you follow this route, the sooner you start the better. If you have had a poor diet and sedentary lifestyle to date, you would be well advised to begin changing your habits before you hit the menopause – or risk possibly suffering worse symptoms.

Change your diet

A healthy diet will help your body to prepare for the menopause and ease it through the natural process. Vitamins A, C and E and the mineral selenium offer protection against heart disease and breast cancer as they neutralise damaging free radicals in the body. Vitamin D, which may be obtained from fortified cereals, margarine, butter and eggs, will aid the absorption of calcium. It's also produced by sunlight so make the most of sunny days whenever you can. Essential fatty acids (EFAs) also help. These are derived from fish oils, oily fish, cooking oils such as rapeseed, sunflower, sesame and corn, as well as evening primrose oil, polyunsaturated-rich soft margarine, green leafy vegetables, game meats, eggs and turkey. Vitamin E will help with hot flushes as it tones the blood vessels.

Avoid excessive consumption of salt and salty foods, sugar and sugary products, as well as caffeine-loaded tea, coffee, cola and chocolate. Also, limit your intake of saturated animal fats by avoiding foods cooked in fat and eating leaner cuts of meat and reduced-fat dairy products.

Natural preparations and supplements

There are many natural preparations available that can also influence menopausal symptoms. Naturally occurring oestrogen can be found in soya

products, rhubarb, linseed, green and yellow vegetables such as celery and
fennel, ginseng and the herb dong quai. A low-fat diet will help, especially if
supplemented with lots of linseeds, nuts, seeds and oily fish. As well as the
high-calcium diet mentioned previously, you could also consider taking a non-
hormonal supplement containing calcium, calcitonin and bisphosphonates. If
in doubt, it may be worthwhile talking to a nutritionist. See also Chapter 10.

Exercise
Finally, don't forget to combine your healthy diet with regular exercise. The
fitter you are, the better you will cope with any physical and psychological
problems. Weight-bearing exercise (see page 98) is particularly important, as it
will help to strengthen the bones and reduce the risk of osteoporosis.

The male menopause
Does the male menopause exist? Yes, or something like it, I would suggest. In
middle age there is a natural decline in the activity of the male hormone
testosterone. When this occurs, some men may experience irritability, lack of
sexual desire and ability, aching joints, dry skin, insomnia, excessive sweating
and depression. This hormonal decline may also affect hair loss.

Some doctors believe that men can benefit by increased levels of testosterone,
in the form of patches or injections. This treatment is quite controversial, as
increased testosterone levels have been linked to both prostate and testicular
cancer. Again, improving your diet and lifestyle is a safer alternative that will
help to alleviate many of the symptoms.

The muscular system
Most of us assume that as we grow older we will experience more aches and
pains in our joints and muscles. Certainly if muscles are not used enough, they
tend to stiffen and weaken, become smaller and dehydrated. A sedentary
lifestyle also means that muscles start to gather fat and the actual muscle mass
reduces with age, mainly due to this decrease in activity. Again, this can lead to
problems with other parts of the body, in terms of support and longevity. You
should not simply assume that you have to accept aches and pains as
inevitable. You can do something about it now.

Rheumatism
It is easy to describe most aches and pains in the joints as rheumatism,
especially as we get older. But the causes may be psychological or physical – or
both. A change in circumstances (promotion, starting a new job, even a new

relationship) can create tension in the muscles, especially when tired or anxious. Unaccustomed, repetitive activity will also cause aching and stiffness of joints, especially the following day.

Even the weather can have a say when it comes to our aches and pains. However, it isn't the weather itself that actually causes the problem: it is that most people will be more aware of their aches and pains when it is especially cold and damp.

If this is your problem, try treating yourself by applying localised heat – it will relax muscular and mental tension. Try heat lamps, heated pads, hot water bottles or a warm bath. Massaging the affected area will relieve tight, aching muscles and can be very relaxing. Anti-inflammatory creams can be used to aid recovery. Of course, if you can afford it, you can always arrange your holidays to escape winter and grab some extra sunshine to prolong your summer.

Arthritis

The most common forms of arthritis are osteoarthritis and rheumatoid arthritis. With osteoarthritis, the joint cartilages become worn down, through wear and tear, causing pain as the bones of the joint rub together. By its very nature, it tends to afflict older people, usually starting in the forties or fifties. Rheumatoid arthritis is characterised by painful inflammation in the joints and may attack any age group. It is caused by the body recognising a 'foreign' body in the joint (usually a piece of tissue) and setting up an attack against it. The pain can be quite severe and is usually accompanied with some swelling and stiffness.

Painkillers and anti-inflammatory tablets and creams can help both types of arthritis in the short term, but you may require medication that can only be obtained on prescription. Resting the joint will also help as will support bandages. Seeing a physiotherapist to identify and treat the joint or muscle will also be worthwhile. Ice and ultra-sound treatment can help to bring faster relief. Your doctor may refer you to a specialist or physiotherapist. Joints can be treated with steroids to calm down the inflammation or fluid removed to ease any swelling. In severe cases surgery may be required to improve the surface of the joint or even replace it, usually very successfully.

Gout

This painful condition is more common in men than women. It is caused by a build-up of uric acid in the blood and can make joints extremely painful, usually in the extremities such as the toes. Diet and lifestyle can play an important part in the prevention and treatment of various forms of arthritis and gout, and your doctor may well point you in the direction of a dietician or nutritionist.

The urinary system

Each of us has two kidneys. The primary function of the kidneys is to filter waste products, excess sodium and water from the blood. The kidneys also help to regulate blood pressure and red blood cell production.

Each kidney is connected to the bladder by a tube (the urethra). With the help of muscle action, urine passes through this tube into the bladder. Urine accumulates in the bladder, which is expandable and gradually increases in size to accommodate the increasing volume of urine. When the bladder eventually fills, nerve signals are sent to the brain, conveying the need to urinate. When the message from the brain signals that it's okay to proceed, urine then drains from the bladder through the urethra, out of the body.

Normal, healthy urine should be clear and of a pale colour. Concentrated urine is deep yellow and may have a strong smell. Food pigments can make the urine red, and drugs can produce a variety of colours. Unless caused by food or drugs, colours other than yellow are abnormal. Cloudy urine should also be investigated: it suggests a urinary tract infection or crystals of salts from uric or phosphoric acid that can build up on the inner surfaces of the kidneys, possibly leading to kidney stones.

Any sign of blood in the urine should be checked immediately by your doctor.

Routine urine analysis includes chemical tests to detect protein, sugar, and ketones, so as to identify diabetes or kidney infections and microscopic examination to detect red and white blood cells. Most tests use a 'dipstick' or thin strip of plastic, impregnated with chemicals that react with substances in the urine and change colour. Dipsticks are routinely used in urinalysis.

Kidney and urinary disorders

Like everything else, these become more common as we grow older. Symptoms vary according to the particular disorder and the part of the system affected.

Fever and nausea are common symptoms, although a bladder infection (cystitis) generally doesn't cause fever. Burning pain while urinating and an urgent need to urinate, which may result in almost constant painful straining, are typical symptoms of bladder infections. The amount of urine is usually small, but bladder control may be lost if a person doesn't urinate immediately. A bacterial infection of the kidney usually causes high fever.

Most people urinate about four to six times a day, mostly in the daytime. Frequent urination without an increase in the total daily amount of urine is a symptom of a bladder infection or of something irritating the bladder. This may be some sort of foreign body, such as a stone, or, much rarer cases, a tumour.

Frequent urination during the night may occur in the early stages of kidney disease, although the cause may simply be drinking a large amount of fluid, especially alcohol, coffee, or tea, late in the evening. Frequent urination at night can also be common in people who have heart or liver problems, or diabetes, even though they don't have any urinary tract disease.

Embarrassing leaks

Many people, as they become older, suffer from a condition called stress incontinence. This is particularly common in women. With age, or as a result of the effects of childbirth, the pelvic muscles lose their strength and the neck of the bladder starts to sag, so that the valves that control the bladder and urinary passage are put under strain. Laughing, coughing, sneezing or lifting increases pressure on the abdomen and can result in urine leakage. However, there are a number of exercises you can do to strengthen your pelvic floor muscles.

First, every time you need pass urine, try stopping in mid-stream. With practice, this should become easy. Even if you're not on the loo, simply tensing the same muscles will help to strengthen them – you can do it quite unobtrusively at any time.

Secondly, stand with your knees bent and feet slightly apart. Tense your pelvic muscles and rotate your hips in a circular motion. Do this for a couple of minutes one way and then change direction.

Third, lie on your back with your knees bent. Contract your front and back passages tightly and hold for a few seconds. Repeat five or six times.

If you keep practising these exercises, your pelvic floor muscles should gradually strengthen and will help to reduce urine leakage in the future.

Incontinence

An uncontrollable loss of urine (incontinence) can result from a variety of conditions. For example, stress incontinence, when a small quantity of urine may leak out, is quite common in women and may happen when she coughs, laughs, runs, or lifts something heavy. This is due to stretched and weakened pelvic muscles, usually caused during childbirth or by changes that occur when oestrogen levels decrease after menopause. Any obstruction to the outflow from the bladder may cause incontinence whenever the pressure inside the bladder exceeds the force of the obstruction. The bladder doesn't completely empty and this may lead to an infection, making things even worse.

Your sight

It is fair to assume that all our senses deteriorate as we age and your eyes will be less able to focus on close objects as you get older. Reading glasses are normally required once we get into our forties, especially if you are already long-sighted. However, there is no reason why you should not continue to enjoy good eyesight well into your later years. If your sight seems to be failing or you are having any problems with your eyes, it is important to visit your doctor or optician straight away. Many minor conditions can be cleared up if dealt with quickly. But even if you feel that your eyesight is good, it is important to have regular checks by an ophthalmic optician.

Caring for your eyes

Bright sunlight and ultraviolet light can produce a fuzzy haze over ageing eyes, so older people should protect their eyes with good sunglasses or a broad-brimmed hat. Regular checks will show up any potential problems such as cataracts, glaucoma, or corneal infections. All of these are treatable if detected early, but potentially serious if allowed to develop – they could even lead to blindness. Cataracts are a cloudiness of the lens, usually as a result of ageing, but commonly in diabetics. Glaucoma causes an increase in the pressure of the eye. The retina and nerves are damaged and the sight deteriorates. Corneal infections affect the transparent layer covering the front of the eye. It is possible for an optician to spot these and other potential illnesses such as diabetes, eye tumours, hypertension and even multiple sclerosis, with known indicators being detected through examination with an ophthalmoscope. This is entirely painless and involves nothing more traumatic than having a bright light shone into your eyes.

Your hearing

Loss of hearing is thought to be the result of ageing combined with lifelong exposure to environmental noise. Our ears are sensitive organs that, as well as hearing, play an important role in our ability to balance. With age, the auditory nerves die and are not replaced, causing a slow deterioration in our hearing. Another problem is the condition known as tinnitus, which presents itself as noises in the ear, such as a constant ringing or buzzing. In the majority of cases, the cause is never found and although there is no known cure, many sufferers use the sound of a radio, TV or cassette player to mask out the noise in their ears. Headphones are also available that play white noise (a mixture of sounds over a wide range of frequencies). Wearing a hearing aid may also help.

Becoming deaf as you grow older is a very gradual process, and it is usually close family who notice that a person is hard of hearing before they do themselves. My mother refused to believe she was losing her hearing and insisted that when people talked to her properly – face to face – she could hear very well! If you suspect (or are told) you are becoming hard of hearing, your doctor will be able to arrange for you to have a hearing test using an audiogram – a painless testing machine that will show the amount of hearing loss you have. He will also suggest treatment options. Some ear problems can be corrected by surgery, but an older patient may have irreversible nerve damage, in which case a hearing aid may be the only option. These are not the awful, ugly things they used to be: today's hearing aids, which contain a microphone, amplifier and speaker, are amazingly small and unobtrusive.

There are some simple causes of deafness that can be easily treated. Glue ear is the term for a collection of thick mucus in the middle ear. Although common in children, it can also occur in adults, especially after a bad cold when the mucus doesn't drain away properly, thus reducing hearing levels. If your ears actually feel blocked up, another likely cause is a build-up of wax residue. There are over-the-counter treatments that can soften the wax, and then it's worthwhile asking your doctor to check your ears and to syringe out any wax or debris.

If you have had a severe ear infection or inflammation of the inner ear, you may find that you suddenly suffer from vertigo. This disconcerting condition will give you a feeling of being out of balance – unable to walk in a straight line. It is thought to be associated with a virus and may last a few weeks, after which it usually improves. Rest and keeping your head still, avoiding any sudden movements, will help and there are drugs available to relieve the symptoms.

Checking yourself out

The word cancer, when mentioned, can strike fear in anyone's mind – *the big C*. Cancer is defined as the abnormal growth of malignant cells, which can spread around the body, and the condition can become life-threatening if the diseased cells affect vital tissues or organs. However, there is plenty that can be done to reduce your chances of dying. Regular screening (see page 115) can help to minimise risks, however, and although incidence of the disease rises with age, your age won't affect your response to any treatment.

For some conditions, there are national screening programmes available – for others, it's a matter of do-it-yourself. But in every case, cancer experts agree that the important thing is that checks are made regularly and any unusual changes investigated by your GP without delay.

Breast examination

One in five women will suffer a breast disorder at some time, with over 80,000 women visiting their GP each year because of such problems. Most women who experience breast problems tend to make a link with cancer, but in fact

Breast self-examination

- Undress and stand in front of a mirror in a good light. Look carefully at the shape, size and position of your breasts.

- Put your hands on top of your head and look at any differences between the two breasts. Now stretch up your arms and look carefully for any pulling or puckering of the skin.

- Gently squeeze your nipple between your thumb and forefinger. It should return to its normal shape after releasing. Any changes, such as a nipple facing a different direction, a blood-stained discharge or cracking of the skin should be reported.

- Next, check for any lumps or irregularities. Lie on your back with your head on a pillow. Place a folded towel under the shoulder of the side of the breast – this makes it easier to examine.

- Put the arm of the breast you are checking under your head. With your other hand flat and fingers together, feel around the breast using small circular movements.

- Move upwards and then carefully check the top half of your breast, still feeling for any unusual lumps or swellings.

nine out of 10 cases are usually benign. Over the age of 50, women are offered regular mammograms as part of a national screening programme. But the best way to minimise the risk is to become familiar with your breasts and examine them yourself carefully every month (see the panel on page 133).

Lumps and bumps ——————————————————————————

Although it is common to have minor lumps or bumps in your breasts, particularly just before menstruation, in the majority of cases, they are due to benign breast changes, which make the breasts feel generally lumpy, and can occur at any age. They are often closely linked with your periods, with the breasts also feeling tender or becoming painful.

The most common type of lump is a **fibroadenoma**. Caused by an over-development of fibrous tissue, these are harmless, painless lumps that vary in size but are usually round and smooth. In most cases, they stop growing when they reach 2–3 cm (just over an inch) in diameter, and unless they become very large, they don't need to be removed.

Cysts are much more common among women who are in their thirties, forties and fifties. A cyst is a fluid-filled sac, which develops quickly and is often painful. It can be treated immediately by your doctor or specialist, who will use a fine syringe to draw out the fluid. This is a simple procedure and the cyst should soon disappear afterwards. However, a cyst can often reappear, but it can be treated again using the same procedure, or with drugs if it becomes a real problem.

If you find a 'new' lump, consult your GP, who will if necessary refer you to a specialist. They will assess the lump, using ultrasound in women under 35 (whose breasts are too dense for a good mammogram result) or a mammogram for older women. If needed, fluid or cells will also be extracted and then examined.

If a lump is thought to be malignant (cancerous), it will be removed. Also, if the surgeon feels the cancer may have spread to the lymph glands under the armpit, these may be removed as well. The extracted lump will be analysed. If it's malignant then, depending on your age, circumstances and preferences, you will probably be offered the following treatments:

- Radiotherapy, in addition to surgery. This X-ray is applied to the chest to kill off growing cancer cells. It may also be used on the ovaries to stop production of the hormone oestrogen, as high levels are associated with the development of some breast cancers.

- Chemotherapy, which is a combination of anti-cancer drugs.

- Hormone treatment can be used to stop the ovaries producing oestrogen.
- Post-menopausal women may be given Tamoxifen. This drug helps to prevent recurrence of the cancer.

Testicular examination

Just as most women need to regularly check their breasts for lumps, men should also get to know their testicles a little better and get used to looking for any lumps and bumps, tenderness or enlargement. You should examine yourself once a month, preferably while having a bath or shower when the body is warm, soapy and relaxed. Each testicle should be gently rolled between thumb and forefinger to feel for any lumps or swellings.

Benign lumps are quite common and the main types include **hydroceles**, which are a collection of fluid around the testicle; **spermatoceles**, cysts that contain some sperm, and **varicoceles**, which are a kind of varicose vein. All are harmless and don't usually require treatment. If the lump feels detached from the testicle, then it's likely to be one of these. However, if it is actually in the testicle, the likelihood is that it may be cancerous. Disorders of the testes usually cause pain that's severe and felt directly at the site of the problem. Whatever the problem and however it manifests itself, if you suspect something is wrong with your testes, you should always consult your doctor. Testicular cancer has a 95 per cent cure rate if it is caught early enough.

Prostate problems

There is no way you can examine your own prostate but if you have problems, you'll probably notice them pretty quickly. The prostate is a walnut-sized gland that lies at the base of a man's bladder and its job is to produce the fluid in semen. Most men over 60 have an enlarged prostate gland, which they'll know about because it blocks the outflow of urine. They may find that they have to urinate frequently at night, because the blockage is causing urine to back up in the bladder. A hesitating start when urinating, a need to strain, a weak and trickling stream of urine, and dribbling at the end of urination may also indicate an obstructed urethra.

Prostate enlargement is generally painless, but an inflammation of the prostate can cause a vague discomfort or sensation of fullness in the area between the anus and genitals. It is extremely common for older men to experience prostate problems and I would recommend that men over the age of 45 insist on yearly check-ups with their doctor.

Benign prostatic hyperplasis (BPH)

This is a benign enlargement of the prostate and symptoms include a frequent need to urinate, hesitancy in getting started, a weak stream, and pain or burning when urinating. It may be treated with drugs or surgery. These days prostate surgery is very straightforward. Taking zinc is believed to help guard against BPH especially once a man hits the age of 45.

Prostate cancer

This kills four times as many men as cervical cancer kills women – and yet there is as yet no screening programme available for prostate cancer as there is for cervical cancer. There may be similar symptoms to BPH but in the early stages it is almost always symptomless so an early diagnosis is essential and many doctors believe there should be a national screening programme. It is believed that the Western diet may be a factor, so eating a high-fibre, low-fat diet could be one way in which men can protect themselves.

Prostatis

This is an inflammation of the prostate gland. There are various symptoms, including those similar to BPH (see above), plus pain in the lower back, abdomen, testicles, groin and pelvis. It is hard to treat, although drugs, microwave therapy – where the prostate is heated up – and massaging the prostate can help in some cases. Giving up smoking, sticking to a healthy diet and learning to cope with stress are all believed to help men avoid prostatis.

Skin examination

The older you are, the more your skin will have suffered from the damaging effects of pollution and over-exposure to the sun. Skin cancer is becoming more and more common, but it is not difficult to examine yourself – as long as you have a good pair of mirrors to help you – and you should do this at least every three months. Most of us know where our freckles, birthmarks and moles are and it is important to keep an eye on them, watching for any changes in shape, edges, colour or size. If you think that a mole has become larger or more raised, you should make a trip to have it checked by a doctor. Itching is another common early symptom, and there may be feelings of tenderness. Nonetheless, remember that skin cancers are usually painless, so always be suspicious. Melanoma, the deadliest form of skin cancer, is a killer, but it can be treated when detected at an early stage.

CHAPTER 9

ংত ওৃ

Your Immune System

Keeping your immune system in shape will help you maintain your good health.

The immune system is our body's defence against foreign invaders. All our lives we take our immune system for granted and most of the time it operates perfectly, without our being conscious of its presence. A strong immune system is vital for our good health and long life, and is especially important as we get older, when it can become less efficient. When it is not functioning correctly, we become susceptible to all the ailments doing the rounds – colds, flu or fatigue. Viral illnesses, such as chickenpox, cold sores, shingles and glandular fever, can attack us when our immune system is in poor shape. More importantly, when severely weakened, the immune system may be unable to respond to more serious illnesses such as cancer and heart disease.

The immune system is made up from a combination of cells and proteins that work together in our body to protect it from harmful micro-organisms (antigens) such as bacteria, viruses and fungi. The immune system plays an important role in the prevention of cancer, by recognising and destroying cells that grow out of control.

Skin: the first barrier

Our immune system is up and running when we are born. Our skin provides a barrier to infection, while acids in the stomach and enzymes around the body destroy invaders on contact. Antibodies are acquired from the mother while the baby is still in the womb, and later through breast-feeding. New-born babies have a passive immunity system, then further immunity is acquired as the body develops its own sophisticated defence system.

Obviously, the natural process of acquiring our first immunity does carry a risk, as the body encounters 'new' and dangerous germs for the first time, before it has built the antibodies to deal with them. This is why artificial methods of vaccination and immunisation, using known germs in a weakened form or a tiny dose, are used to help the body create its own immunity, without the same inherent dangers.

However, many factors can weaken our immunity. Modern forms of food processing, chemical residues in food and the over-prescription of antibiotics are just some of the factors contributing to the gradual erosion of immunity efficiency today. In addition, our modern lifestyle, with its central heating, air conditioning and atmospheric pollution may also be implicated in our susceptibility to viral illnesses.

So how do we make our immune system work more efficiently in the modern world, especially as we get older? We already know that eating a good, healthy diet and taking regular exercise will help to boost and maintain our immune system, but some things may help more than others. Below I list my top immune system tips that will certainly help to keep the bugs at bay, and especially useful during the winter months.

Learn to breathe correctly

Get an energy fix by breathing correctly. Breathing correctly brings oxygen deep into your lungs and cells, pushing out toxins. This can reduce stress levels, boost your immunity, and even help with depression or sleepless nights. This is because our bodies need to be supplied with the right amount of oxygen, helping to boost our brain and other vital organs with essential nutrients.

We usually take breaths that are too shallow, especially when we are stressed, using only part of our lungs. This leads to a poor exchange of oxygen and CO_2 in the bloodstream, depriving our bodies of these vital gases. When you breathe, you should use your diaphragm, which lies at the bottom of the chest cavity. Use this muscle to breathe in and out without allowing your upper chest to rise and fall. Aim to breathe slowly, smoothly and deliberately, aiming to achieve about ten deep breaths a minute. Practise breathing for a few minutes, holding yourself upright for better air movement. Think about this when walking outside in a clean air environment (the park rather than the street!) to take in the full benefit of your surroundings. Make this a daily habit for the maximum effect, and also regulate your breathing during aerobic exercise, which will help to sustain your energy.

Check your diet

A healthy diet is by far the most effective way of strengthening your immune system. Please do not dismiss the importance of eating at least five portions of fresh fruit and vegetables every day. To prove the point, vegetarians tend to show an increased immune efficiency with a lower risk of heart disease, cancer, high blood pressure, high blood cholesterol and diabetes. It is worth repeating that fresh fruit and vegetables supply concentrated levels of vitamin A, C, E and beta-carotene – antioxidant nutrients that neutralise the potentially harmful effects of too many free radicals, and provide a powerful protective force against cancer and heart disease. They are also a rich source of phyto-chemicals – naturally occurring compounds with cancer-preventative properties. The best fruit and vegetables to boost the immune system include onions, apricots, oranges, mangoes, tomatoes, red (bell) peppers, carrots, spinach and broccoli.

Take echinacea

Many people believe that when it comes to the immune system and natural remedies, nothing beats echinacea. Known as the 'immune herb', echinacea's antibacterial and antiviral properties have made it probably the best-selling natural remedy. It is often used as a natural alternative to antibiotics to treat and reduce the severity of common infections such as colds and flu. Echinacea is claimed to increase immune efficiency, activating the production of the immune system's white blood cells and strengthening the body's ability to resist and fight off viral infections. Available in the form of capsules, concentrated drops, tincture and extracts, echinacea is best taken as a short-term remedy until any infection clears.

Add garlic

Like echinacea, garlic has a reputation as one of nature's miracle cures. Garlic has been used for thousands of years as an antibiotic. It features strong anticoagulant, antiviral and antibacterial properties, and helps to reduce cholesterol, lower blood pressure and thin the blood. Garlic contains many phyto-chemical compounds, including allicin (released when a garlic is cut or crushed), which is believed to be responsible for its wide-ranging therapeutic properties. These compounds are thought to produce powerful antioxidant activity, helping to stimulate the immune system and mop up free radicals. One or two raw cloves of garlic each day will help to boost your immunity, and give protection against colds and flu. If that sounds unappetising (not to say anti-social), there are many forms of garlic supplements that can be taken every day (see Chapter 4 – A Healthy Diet).

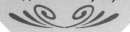
Boost your intake of essential fatty acids

Oily fish should form part of any illness-prevention diet. Three portions of oily fish (sardines, herrings, mackerel, pilchards, salmon and trout) a week will strengthen the immune system, boost its response to disease threats, help to prevent cardiovascular problems and provide a good recipe for long-term good health. Oily fish is a highly concentrated source of omega-3 essential fatty acids, which are polyunsaturated oils closely linked to immune efficiency. Omega-3 essential fatty acid also makes the blood less likely to clot, reducing the risk of a heart attack or stroke. Unlike some fats, omega-3 cannot be manufactured by the body, so it is vital that we get the required amount from our food. Supplements are available for both omega-3 and omega-6.

Take regular exercise

We cannot talk about strengthening our immune system without referring to exercise. Not only does it increase both our energy and vitality, it also helps us feel more relaxed, look good and feel good, and it can add years to our lives. Research shows that just 30 minutes a day of moderate aerobic exercise such as walking, swimming, cycling, etc., can significantly reduce the risk of heart disease, strokes, high blood pressure and diabetes. Regular exercise increases our metabolic rate, protects us from failing memory, reduces pre-menstrual tension and can guard against the onset of osteoporosis. Ignore regular exercise at your peril. (See also Chapter 7 – Keeping Fit).

Smile please

Most of the medical profession would agree that laughter is a good medicine, for research has shown that people who laugh a lot are less likely to suffer from stress-related disorders and high blood pressure. They also recover more quickly from illnesses and usually live longer. How's that for an incentive to be happy! Of course, we can't simply make ourselves happy when circumstances prevent us from doing so, but we can change our outlook to be more positive about many aspects of our lives. Philosophical attitudes to circumstances that we can't change can be very helpful and progressive. Laughing actually stimulates the body into releasing immunoglobins (natural antibodies in the blood that boost the immune system), so that our bodies are better equipped to fight disease. So, when you are happy, smiling or laughing, it really is good for you.

Get plenty of sleep

Undisturbed sleep encourages efficient cell repair and renewal, rejuvenating and revitalising both the body and the mind. Insomniacs are usually more stressed, have less energy and are more likely to suffer from high blood pressure and high blood cholesterol. Stimulants such as coffee, tea, cola, chocolate, spices and alcohol will interfere with the quality of sleep and should be avoided as much as possible, certainly late in the evening. Milky bedtime drinks can be helpful, as they contain tryptophan, an amino acid that stimulates the production of serotonin, a soothing chemical that calms the mind and helps to encourage restful sleep.

Avoid stress

When we are under stress, the body reacts by directing all of its resources to what is known as the 'flight or fight' response, leaving our immune system severely compromised. Stress also depletes our level of vitamin C, an antioxidant that helps to detoxify the body of harmful substances and is vital to the efficient functioning of the immune system. A balanced diet providing B-vitamins and magnesium can help to reduce any stress levels, as does regular exercise. Relaxation and meditation with deep breathing exercises (see page 138, Learn to breathe correctly), as well as aromatherapy and reflexology are also excellent stress-relieving aids. Caffeine can aggravate stress, so cut down on coffee, tea and cola drinks, and replace with calming herbal teas such as camomile, blackberry, blackcurrant, lemon balm, peppermint or fennel.

Drink lots of water

An excess of toxins in the body can cause the lymphatic system to become sluggish, which can result in low energy levels, poor digestion, headaches, allergies, weight gain, skin problems, etc. Although our body will attempt to naturally detoxify toxins through the lymphatic system, it may need a little help to do so and regular flushing through with water will help this process.

Drinking **at least** six glasses of water each day will encourage lymphatic drainage, helping to remove unwanted toxins from the bloodstream and lightening the load of the all-important immune system. Drinking that amount regularly isn't difficult if you plan ahead. Have one glass of water in the morning when you wake up, then have one at breakfast (as well as your tea or coffee, fruit juice, etc.), mid-morning, at lunchtime, mid-afternoon, during the evening, and before going to bed. Add these to your normal tea, coffee, juices, etc., and you'll be creating one of the best habits of a lifetime.

Eat yoghurt

Live yoghurt is claimed to strengthen the immune system. Research in the United States has revealed that live yoghurt containing active cultures can stimulate the production of gamma interferon, a naturally occurring antiviral agent that boosts immune response. Interferon activates the 'fighting' cells within the immune system, making the body more resistant to bacteria, infection and viruses. So it is worthwhile adding live yoghurt to your shopping list. It's great at breakfast, with or without cereal or fruit, and makes an excellent snack.

Use herbal remedies

Herbal remedies have been around for thousands of years. Natural herbs contain a number of active ingredients that can help to improve your health. They can provide gentle aids to the normal functioning of the body, and also act in a preventative capacity. The list below gives a few that can aid the immune system, or treat causes that will affect the immune system, such as stress.

Some herbal remedies can have side-effects, so it is important to talk to a herbalist or your doctor, especially if you are taking other medication.

Aloe vera

A very popular herb which comes from the cactus family. Can be used as a laxative as well as for digestive complaints. Better known for treating cuts, burns, grazes and sunburn, and to be found in many creams and ointments. Aloe vera is said to be good for the skin, asthma and arthritis.

Camomile

Makes a delicious and delicate alternative to tea, improves digestion and helps in cases of stress, anxiety or depression. Also used for eczema, gum disease, mouth ulcers and insomnia. Is sometimes used to reduce bowel inflammation.

Factors that will damage your immune system's efficiency

- Alcohol depresses vitamin B and zinc levels that play an important role in our immune system. Alcohol can also reduce the uptake of other important nutrients.

- Cigarette smoking can raise the white blood cell count, de-activating the immune system. Smoking can also lead to chronic bronchitis and lung cancer.

- Repeated use of drugs such as steroids or antibiotics to treat infections can destroy beneficial bacteria in the gut that play an important defensive role.

- Deficiencies of many nutrients, especially proteins, vitamins and minerals, will make the immune system less efficient.

- Prolonged stress reduces the effectiveness of the immune system.

- Don't overdo exercise – regular exercise will boost your immune system but excessive exercise can depress it.

- Lack of natural daylight is associated with a greater level of illness and infection.

Evening primrose

Evening primrose oil is used to combat eczema, pre-menstrual tension and diabetes and to lower blood cholesterol. The active ingredient is gamma linolenic acid, which has anti-inflammatory properties. Recent research, although not conclusive, shows that this herb may have some anti-cancer activity.

Ginger

Ginger can help to improve digestion and reduce flatulence. Ginger is an excellent herb for helping to improve circulation and lowering blood pressure and therefore benefits the heart. It can be drunk as a herbal remedy during colds and flu to promote perspiration and reduce temperature during fevers.

Ginkgo biloba

A popular herb used in Chinese medicine. Helps to ease depression, memory loss and brain disorders such as Alzheimer's. It has antioxidant properties, which are known to boost circulation and nerve action.

Ginseng

Well-known for reducing stress and tiredness, it has been used as an energy booster in Chinese medicine for thousands of years. It is also thought to improve both intellectual and memory performance.

Green tea

Green tea is a rich source of flavonoid antioxidants, which reduce the effects of damaging free radicals and oxidants. Clinical studies also suggest that green tea reduces blood cholesterol, lowers blood pressure and acts as an anti-clotting agent.

Milk thistle

Used as a boost for the liver and to treat hepatitis, alcohol-related liver disease, cirrhosis, gallstones and psoriasis. Milk thistle is known as a popular hangover prevention and cure as it is supposed to regenerate liver cells and reduce the effects of alcohol.

St John's wort

Recommended for the treatment of depression and anxiety, and may have some antiviral activity. Contains hypericin, which boosts the levels of serotonin, helping to control sleep, eating disorders and mood levels.

CHAPTER 10

Natural Therapies

When the term 'alternative medicine' was first used, most of us were suspicious of the many strange treatments that were on offer. Also the conventional medical experts were less than convinced, often dismissing alternative medicine as unscientific or even dangerous. Although alternative, or complementary, therapy has been around far longer than conventional medicine, at one time there were no ruling bodies to monitor the activities of practitioners. Consequently some unscrupulous characters set themselves up in practice taking advantage of those seeking help, and not helping to enhance the reputation of natural treatments. Fortunately those days are mostly gone and the majority of therapies have their own ruling bodies, with guidelines and training programmes along with a strict code of ethics.

Today, alternative or complementary medicines, or natural therapies, have become a respected part of the health sector. Many doctors, clinics and hospitals now acknowledge that many types of natural therapies have a place alongside orthodox medicine – many doctors have become natural therapists in their own right, or will refer patients to qualified therapists, working in the same surgery or clinic.

Qualifications

Unless you are being advised to see a natural therapist through the recommendation of your doctor, it is worth contacting the governing body to find out the nearest

Properly administered complementary therapies can have health benefits for the over 50s.

qualified registered practitioners (see the list on page 203). They will usually also be happy to provide detailed information about their particular therapy if you send them a self-addressed stamped envelope.

When selecting a practitioner, check the standard of qualification, how many years they have been practising, and how much is the price of the treatment, including the initial consultation. Once you have made your decision, it is worth having a preliminary chat with the therapist or practitioner, explaining why you think you may need the treatment and to see if the therapist has any experience in treating similar conditions in other patients. You should also ask how long a therapy course is likely to take before any improvement will normally be felt, so that once you start, you can judge whether the treatment is being successful or not.

Major therapies

During my years of editing *Good Health* magazine, we had hundreds of readers telling their own stories about how a particular natural therapy had solved their health problems. Whether the actual treatment did the trick or not, there can be no doubt that as far as our readers were concerned, it had changed many of their lives for ever.

On pages 147–55, I have listed in alphabetical order most of the popular therapies that I think may prove particularly useful to the over 50s, with a brief description of their origins, the treatment and what ailments it is usually used for. It is only meant as a rough guide. Please contact the associations listed at the end of this book for more details about specific therapies.

Do remember that although natural therapies and remedies have a place in promoting good health, they are not a substitute for conventional medicine. Any worrying symptoms should always be checked by your doctor, to ensure that they do not relate to a serious complaint that requires conventional treatment or surgery.

You should also inform your doctor before embarking on any course of complementary therapy, especially if you are already having treatment or being prescribed any drugs. Not all therapies are suitable for everyone – ask your doctor if you are in any doubt. In many cases your doctor may recommend a particular therapist who has dealt successfully with other patients.

Acupuncture

This ancient Eastern art of healing dates back more than 2,000 years. Traditional acupuncture is based on the belief that our health is dependent on the balanced functioning of the body's energy. This is governed by the flow of energy (*chi*) along meridians or channels throughout the body. When there is a disturbance in the energy flow, ill-health can occur. Acupuncture is said to restore health through insertion of fine needles into particular points just beneath the skin. Gentle manipulation disperses any stagnant energy and restores the normal energy balance of the body. When inserted, the fine needles rarely cause any bleeding.

An initial diagnosis can take up to an hour and you will be asked details about your particular problem and your medical history. Acupuncturists will often examine your tongue and assess your pulse at a variety of places on the body.

Common ailments successfully treated include pain, anxiety, eczema, hay fever, asthma, migraine, high blood pressure and menstrual disorders.

Acupressure
Acupressure uses the same points on the meridian lines as acupuncture, but they are stimulated by the application of gentle finger pressure rather than needles (see also Massage and Reflexology).

Alexander Technique
The Alexander Technique is a method of re-educating people to make them more aware of how they move, sit and hold themselves. Over a lifetime we can develop bad habits of posture and movement, which can tend to make us look older. Often our posture while undertaking everyday tasks puts unnecessary strain on the body – for example, the way we sit at a desk or even answer the telephone, the way we walk or hold ourselves. A practitioner will work with a client to identify habitual misuse of the muscles and demonstrate how to change these habits – an instant way of removing a few years.

The Alexander Technique is an excellent way of learning how to adopt a good posture, therefore helping to promote better health. It may be taught in classes or in a one-to-one situation, although the latter is obviously more expensive.

Conditions such as stiff necks, shoulder tension, back pain and headaches can all be relieved by using the Alexander Technique. It can also be used to treat anxiety, insomnia, digestive disorders and pains in muscles and joints.

Aromatherapy
Aromatherapy uses essential oils, extracted from various plants, to improve physical and emotional well-being. Applied using either massage, through inhalation or in a bath, the aroma from the oil can positively affect a person's mood and help with physical ailments.

An aromatherapist will usually ask you questions about medical history, general health and lifestyle before deciding which oils are most appropriate for you.

Treatment of stress-related illness such as depression or anxiety can respond well to this treatment as the sessions are relaxing and can help to ease away aches and tension. Many healthcare professionals also train in aromatherapy and use it in various aspects of nursing – maternity, intensive care, coronary care, rheumatology, elderly care, cancer and hospice care. Aromatherapy is used primarily to ease pain and relieve tension, helping a patient to sleep and thus reducing the need for conventional drugs.

Aromatherapy oils can also be used purely for pleasure. Many chemists and health shops sell popular essential oils that can be used at home in your bath or heated by candle in a special container. Some of the scents are sensual and can be used to enhance a romantic evening or to simply create an atmosphere of well-being. There are many aromas to choose from and the labels will specify what they are usually used for. Always buy 100 per cent essential oils and follow the instructions for use carefully.

Ayurveda

Ayurveda, the ancient art of Indian healing, means 'science of life' and, having been around for over 3,000 years, is one of the oldest systems of healthcare but it is only recently that there has been a dramatic surge of interest in it.

Ayurveda is a holistic system that encourages mental, spiritual and emotional well-being. According to Ayurvedic philosophy, retaining health and vitality depends on three energies which are called *doshas*, each having their own name – *Vata*, *Pitta* and *Kapha*. Each dosha is a combination of two elements – *Vata* is associated with the air element (also called *ether*), *Pitta* is primarily a fire element but with water too, and *Kapha* is a combination of both earth and water. Each of us has a unique combination of doshas, and the aim of Ayurveda is to bring them into a better balance and then learn to keep them in harmony to sustain our well-being.

An Ayurveda practitioner will establish your dosha, based on your physical build and health history, as well as lifestyle habits, ranging from diet to relationships. A treatment plan will usually recommend some dietary and lifestyle adjustments, a selection of ayurvedic herbs, plus a daily regime involving yoga or meditation. You may also be offered an internal and detox programme called *panchakarma*, which involves enemas or laxatives. The most enjoyable part of your Ayurveda treatment will be a massage, which can involve two masseurs, one standing on each side of you, working on your energy points to stimulate the free flow of *pran* around your body.

Bach Flower Remedies

These remedies were developed in the 1930s by Dr Edward Bach, based on the belief that a healthy mind is the key to a healthy body. The system first used 38 healing plants (today there are many more) to treat negative emotions, and all are administered by diluting drops of liquid in a small glass of water. Some remedies include a mixture of plants to help people cope with everyday pressures.

The flower remedies can be bought over the counter from most chemists and health shops. They include treatments for mood swings and anxiety, nervous disorders, emotional or mental shock.

Chinese medicine

Traditional Chinese medicine has been around for nearly 4,000 years and is still the most widely practised system of medicine in the world. It is based on the idea that any symptom is part of an overall disharmony in the body. The cause of the disharmony must be classified through interpretation of the *yin* and *yang* elements of the body, and treated with herbal remedies. *Yang* organs are thought to 'channel' energy with reference to acute pain and headaches, and *yin* organs 'hold' energy, referring to dull aches, pains and tiredness. The skill of the practitioner is to identify which is influencing the patient.

Before beginning treatment, a practitioner will assess a patient's overall health. Once a diagnosis has been reached, a herb formula will be prescribed, which will be formulated in tea, pills, tablets or powders. Chinese medicine can be used to treat many ailments but is particularly known for helping in the treatment of skin disorders such as eczema, infertility and menstrual problems, as well as digestive complaints, respiratory illness and fatigue.

Chiropractic

This is a system of manual manipulation specially designed to treat mechanical disorders of joints, particularly the spine, thus affecting the whole nervous system. Practitioners believe that when the body's systems are in harmony, the body will have the ability to help heal itself from within. Any impediment to the normal nerve supply caused by slight misalignments can cause pain, discomfort or even disease and needs to be corrected in order to effect full recovery.

Chiropractors can treat a number of conditions including back pain, sciatica, tension headaches, migraine, neck, shoulder and arm pains, sports injuries and strains. This type of therapy is suitable for people of all ages.

Colonic hydrotherapy

Colonic hydrotherapy (or irrigation) consists of introducing warm purified water into the colon under low pressure, via a small tube. When the colon is full the water is allowed to flow out through a larger tube, taking with it any loose debris. This process is carried out a number of times during one treatment, which lasts around 40 minutes. The treatment is not painful but patients may feel a slight discomfort, such as having diarrhoea. Modesty is preserved throughout the treatment.

Conditions that benefit from colonic hydrotherapy include constipation, diarrhoea, irritable bowel syndrome, candida and diverticulitis.

Craniosacral therapy

This gentle therapy uses no manipulation – just a very light touch. By placing their hands on the skull and different areas of the body, therapists 'listen to' and detect stresses, tensions, or traumas that may have been stored in the body. Once they have been identified, the body is then able to let the restrictions go and return to a balanced 'craniosacral motion', relieving any pain and symptoms.

Craniosacral therapy is so mild that it is suitable for people of all ages including those in fragile or acutely painful conditions. It is said that it can aid people with most ailments by encouraging a self-healing process.

Feng shui

Feng shui is an ancient art of arranging living and working space to bring physical and spiritual harmony to your home – or office. Feng shui seeks to harmonise the flow of *chi* (life energy) within a living space to enhance the health, wealth and happiness of those who live or work there. It is taken very seriously in the Far East and many Western companies are obliged to acknowledge feng shui rules when designing their buildings or offices.

A consultant will visit your home and recommend specific furniture positions, colour schemes, plants, ornaments, or even the siting of the front door! You can help the flow of *chi* yourself by removing clutter from rooms and surfaces and making sure that there is plenty of space around beds and furniture. Healthy plants (but not sharp-leafed ones) are believed to attract *chi* and can counterbalance electromagnetic fields around televisions or computers. Mirrors should be carefully positioned (usually inside wardrobes) so that they don't reflect *chi* and disturb energy patterns.

Herbal medicine

Herbal medicine goes back over 4,000 years and uses both herb and plant remedies. Practitioners use a holistic approach to rebalance the body by using specific plants which have a particular affinity with certain organs or systems, restoring health and allowing the body to fight off disease.

When you first go to a herbalist, they will take notes of your medical history. Treatment may then include advice about diet and lifestyle as well as any suggested plant remedies. The most common ailments treated are skin problems, digestive disorders, angina, varicose veins, arthritis, insomnia and stress, plus allergies such as hay fever and asthma. It is worth noting that the modern pharmaceutical industry is actively studying plants to use their ingredients in today's drugs.

Homeopathy

This form of medicine has been around for more than 150 years and works on the principle of treating like with like. For instance, if a healthy person is given a homeopathic remedy such as belladonna berries, it will produce symptoms similar to scarlet fever. If the belladonna berries are given in a minute dose to a patient with scarlet fever, in many cases, it will help to cure the condition.

Before prescribing a remedy, a practitioner will take into account the patient's temperament, personality, characteristics and reaction to their environment.

Remedies contain minute amounts of natural substances, in the form of liquids, powders, tablets or pills. Homeopathy can help in the treatment of a wide range of problems, including acne, allergies, asthma, arthritis, back pain, eczema, insomnia, migraine, menopausal problems and rheumatism.

Hydrotherapy

Therapeutic bathing is one of the oldest natural therapies. Having lost favour for a while, it has recently re-emerged as a favourite. There are many different ways of using water in therapy treatment. Different temperatures can be applied to the body through methods of application that include baths, showers, ice packs, compresses and steam. The water can also be used to dissolve different forms of medication so that they can be absorbed through the skin (as in aromatherapy). Special exercises may also be carried out in water, which provides both support and resistance, making it suitable for weaker people with inflamed joints or muscles. Water applied to the body under gentle pressure can also provide lymphatic circulation. Moist heat when applied directly with a hot compress can relieve pain and improve circulation. Hydrotherapy may also be used to detoxify the skin and promote a feeling of well-being.

If you have any health problems, especially diabetes or circulatory disorders, or you are frail, then check with your doctor before embarking on a hydrotherapy session.

Hypnotherapy

Contrary to popular belief, hypnotherapy will not put you into a trance or make you do things you don't want to do. It is actually a state of altered awareness, which can only be achieved with the help of a trained practitioner. It is thought that through this awareness a patient can tap into their subconscious and deal with unwanted thoughts or behavioural patterns.

A hypnotherapist should take a detailed personal history before helping a patient to use their mind to achieve a relaxed and suggestive state.

Hypnotherapy is used to help many types of phobia, lack of confidence, insomnia, anxiety, depression and unwanted habits such as smoking or weight gain. It can also be used to treat skin diseases, asthma and migraine.

Iridology

Clear, shining eyes have been associated with good health for hundreds of years. The iris, which is the coloured part of the eye surrounding the pupil, is made up of thousands of nerve endings that are connected to the brain via the hypothalamus. Iridology involves studying a person's eyes in order to make a diagnosis. The practitioner produces an iris 'map', which charts out the reflex zones in relation to the body's systems. For example, the left iris reflects information on the left side of the body while the right iris reflects the right side. The structure and basic colours of the irises, including the spots, flecks and streaks, reveal an individual's strengths and weaknesses and any conditions within the body, enabling the iridologist to reach a diagnosis. Eye colour is believed to be linked to our constitution. People with blue eyes are said to be prone to arthritis and those with brown eyes have a slow metabolic rate. People with mixed irises may be prone to weak digestion. Iridology is sometimes used as an additional diagnostic tool by homeopaths and naturopaths.

Kinesiology

This particular therapy gently tests the muscles in the body to gain an analysis of the balance and imbalances of the body's system. After a consultation to take an in-depth profile of the patient's health, the kinesiologist then applies gentle pressure to the patient's outstretched arm while placing suspect foods and substances close to the body, and asks them to push back with equal pressure. When a therapist detects a possible allergy or intolerance, the client's arm becomes weak. Balance is restored with a combination of movements, flower remedies, supplements and dietary advice.

Kinesiology takes a holistic approach and is used to treat muscular aches and pains, fatigue, anxiety, mood swings, depression, fears or phobias, allergies and nutritional deficiencies.

Kinesiology – a personal account

When our daughter was 15, she seemed to be generally unwell, although she had no obvious symptoms apart from a constant lethargy. Neither our doctor nor the local hospital could find anything wrong with her, so after two years my wife and I turned to a kinesiologist. He diagnosed that she was allergic to some foods, particularly wheat, tomatoes and mushrooms – and at the time her favourite food was pizza! We put her on an exclusion diet and she was back to her old self in a matter of weeks.

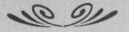

Massage

A trained massage therapist uses special techniques to relieve muscle tension and stiff or aching joints, improve the circulation and help the body to eliminate any waste products. After a good massage, your skin will develop a healthy glow, and the relaxation felt afterwards can be of benefit from both a mental and physical perspective.

Massage is one of the few therapies that can be tried at home. A general body massage from a friend or partner can help to improve health and a feeling of well-being. Used in conjunction with massage oil or aromatherapy essential oils (see Aromatherapy), various techniques can be used and massage oil will help the hand to glide over the skin and help knead the flesh. Slow strokes are relaxing and a brisker action can be used a more invigorating effect, helping to improve circulation.

Naturopathy

This is a system of healing that works by promoting the body's ability to heal itself. Naturopaths believe that good health depends on adopting a healthy and well-balanced lifestyle. Naturopathy uses a combination of treatments such as diet control, in some cases fasting, as well as hydrotherapy, manipulation, exercise and even psychology. During a consultation, the practitioner will ask questions about the patient's life and medical history before embarking on a course of therapy tailored to the individual. Naturopaths believe that any medicine given should be gentle in action and chosen with regard to the whole person and not just a particular illness.

Many conditions can be treated with naturopathy, including irritable bowel syndrome, skin complaints, digestive, respiratory or circulatory disorders, hormonal difficulties and joint problems such as arthritis. Alternatively, a naturopath can be consulted by a patient who doesn't have any specific symptoms but just wants to lead a healthier lifestyle.

Nutritional therapy —————————————————————————

Nutritional therapy aims to identify health problems that have been caused by biological factors. Many people develop health disorders through a poor diet. The practitioner will usually take very detailed information about the patient's lifestyle, eating habits and their previous medical history before investigating possible problems such as allergies, nutritional deficiencies, toxic overload or poor digestion. Once a diagnosis is reached, a diet and supplement regime is developed to redress the balance and allow the body to heal itself. Nutritional therapy does not claim to be a miracle cure but is more a process of exploration. However, it has been found to be a successful way of treating digestive disorders, migraine, lethargy, weight gain and sinus problems.

Osteopathy ————————————————————————————————

This well-known treatment is a system of medicine relating to the relationship between the musculo-skeletal system of the body and the way in which it functions. It is used to ease pain and enable the body's frame to work as efficiently as possible. Osteopaths work with their hands using different techniques that involve varying levels of manipulation, depending on the patient. Soft manipulation is reserved for children and the elderly.

This treatment is sometimes available on the NHS, although patients will need to be referred by their doctor. It is used to help back pain, tension headaches and joint strain, as well as migraines and dizziness.

Psychotherapy and counselling ————————————————————

Psychotherapy and counselling are used to help heal the mind by talking to another person. Problems to be treated include depression, grief, shock, even long-term decisions such as a career change or moving on after a failed marriage. Sessions may be one-to-one or may take place in a group where people can help to ease their emotions by sharing their experiences with others who are in similar situations. Psychotherapy tends to be a longer-term and expensive process, so it would be worthwhile talking to your doctor first. In any case, you should get a referral from your doctor so that the counsellor or psychotherapist is aware of any problems that you may have.

Reflexology

Reflexology is an ancient science dating from the time of the Ancient Egyptians. Using thumbs and fingers, practitioners apply direct pressure to precise areas on the reflex points in the soles of the feet, working through the nerve pathways of the body to create an energy release. It is thought that reflexology stimulates the centre of the brain, which then releases endorphins, the body's natural painkillers, bringing relief to many ailments.

This gentle therapy can be used to help a variety of conditions but is particularly successful with migraine, asthma, hay fever, constipation, bowel complaints, hypertension and back pain. As reflexology is non-invasive, it is safe to use on the elderly and terminally ill as a relaxation treatment.

Shiatsu

Japanese 'finger pressure' therapy works on similar principles to acupuncture, but instead of needles, practitioners use their thumbs, fingers, elbows and sometimes even knees and feet to apply pressure to the body's meridians, or energy lines. The aim of this therapy is to stimulate the circulation, helping to release toxins and tension from the muscles, leaving patients feeling calm, relaxed and with a sense of well-being. Shiatsu can be used to treat headaches, migraines, respiratory illnesses, insomnia, anxiety and depression, digestive disorders, bowel troubles, menstrual problems, back pain and rheumatic and arthritic complaints.

CHAPTER 11

Relationships and Sex

Being able to handle your relationship effectively will reduce your stress levels.

That word 'relationships' does tend to imply that this chapter is aimed solely at couples. However, it is true to say that much of what I am about to say will apply just as well to other relationships, with friends, siblings and so on. So don't skip over this chapter because you're single – you will find plenty here that applies to you too.

By the time we reach our fifties, we will all have experienced a large number of relationships with all sorts of people over the preceding decades. And how we deal with other people in our lives has a profound effect on our well-being, both mental and physical. Relationships can make life worth living or they can literally make you ill – and at least part of the outcome is down to you. The better you handle your relationships, the less stressful your life will be, so take a look at the people in your life and how you deal with them.

Problems with partners

You could be forgiven for thinking that most problems for couples start at around the age of 50 years, for it always seems that there are more separated or divorced middle-aged people around us as we become older. However, don't think that because you've hit 50, your relationship with your partner is about to go down the pan: the chances are that at least half of those people who have separated or divorced did so when they were younger. Statistics produced by the General Register Office in the UK show that most divorces occur with people in their mid- to late thirties, with the average length of a marriage now being around 15 years.

Nowadays, one in three marriages ends in divorce, which is acknowledged to be one of the most stressful life events there is. Strangely, it doesn't seem to put people off getting married. Most divorcees will marry again – usually to another divorcee. Increasingly, modern younger couples are not getting married at all, preferring to live together, although even co-habitees still tend to get married at a later date when they are in their early thirties. Compare this to your mother and father, or your grandmother and grandfather, and you will quickly see that marriages or relationships used to last a lot longer than they do today.

So are we better or worse off than previous generations? It's worth remembering that 50 years ago roles for both men and women were clearly defined, with men going out to work and women usually staying at home to look after the children and home. This was a full-time and demanding task without the luxury of labour-saving devices such as washing machines, dishwashers, tumble dryers or refrigerators, which are today considered necessities. There were also fewer opportunities to create new friendships, and socialising revolved around the family, with relatives tending to live in the same community and locality. And just because a couple were together for many years, it doesn't necessarily mean they were happy. It simply meant that marriage then was for life – good or bad – and expectations were not as high as they are in today's world.

Today's relationships for couples may not last so long, but they are far more complex. With the modern family unit being more flexible in terms of work and geographic location, the support network of immediate family has become less available to the modern couple, who themselves may or may not be married. And it is the first of those modern couples, now getting into their fifties, who are finding that they have their own individual concerns, which may make it hard for them to give enough attention to their relationship with their partner. Men are usually wrapped up in their work and careers, while the majority of women will be trying to juggle the demands of work, the home, the menopause, not to mention attending to both children and ageing parents. If one partner goes through a period of personal growth or change, the other may feel threatened. Since most couples are usually aged within five years of each other, they may tend to experience the physical stresses of middle age at around the same time, too, making life even more difficult.

Sexual problems ─────────────────────────────────────

If you have been in the same relationship since you were in your twenties, sexual incompatibilities may become an issue for the first time now, with boredom, tiredness or routine all taking their toll. Either one – or both – of you may be worried about your attractiveness or there may be physical problems such as impotence or lack of vaginal lubrication. Women may become dissatisfied and men feel threatened or incompetent. Not surprisingly, there is a danger of a crisis reaction, such as having an affair, the results of which can be extremely stressful and destabilising for everyone.

But all is not doom and gloom. Most couples survive the difficult patches and many end up closer than they were before, with more time for each other, especially after any children have left home. Growth and change can be stimulating and may bring new interests for both partners. Love-making, although possibly less frequent, may become more loving, enjoyable and carefree. Age brings both love and tenderness, which can bring couples even closer together.

Making the effort

Everyone needs to put some effort into preserving their relationships, especially when many changes are taking place. It is important to set some time aside for each other every day to discuss the day's problems or simply catch up.

Make sure that you actually listen to your partner and let them know that you have listened and understood. This is not the same as waiting for them to finish talking so that you can reply, which can often be the case with couples who have known each other for many years. Even if you disagree with your partner's viewpoint, respect his or her opinions and try to see the problems from both sides. Be true to your feelings and express them to your partner without getting angry or losing your temper.

Most importantly, never take your partner for granted, and always make an effort to show your appreciation of your relationship. This includes giving each other separate space and time occasionally, while still sharing some activities so that you have joint experiences. Remind yourself of all the good things about your partner and make a unexpected gesture of love or affection now and then – perhaps a romantic evening, a small gift, a surprise show or weekend away. Even a bunch of flowers will always be appreciated. Spontaneous thought really counts for a lot in most relationships.

A good relationship thrives on continued thought and effort from both partners, and should never be taken for granted, especially when everything else has become routine and comfortable. Be determined to keep your interests and enthusiasm and continue to live life to the full, both together and individually.

Problems with your children

If your children are still at home they will probably be going through their teenage years, which can put a strain on any relationship. Much has been written and said about helping teenagers through what is, without doubt, the most difficult time of growing up. But it is worth remembering that you have a life and feelings too. This is a time when children really start to want to 'fly the nest' and they will tend to dislike everything about their home and parents, without even knowing why. It's important to be sensitive to their moodiness and emotions but it's often best to allow them to take their course without too much interference. It's also important that you make it clear that you expect some degree of respect – if you don't ask for it, you won't get it!

Teenagers prefer and frequently demand time on their own – so let them have it. Set down some general parameters for their protection, preferably with their (grudging) agreement and then allow them to run their own lives. They will learn, through experience, to use their independence wisely, and you will have the satisfaction of knowing that they are discovering what it is to be adult. Of course, I'm not suggesting that you leave them entirely to their own devices – you should maintain some level of control, but start to reduce it gradually. Both parties should benefit from the freedom of this arrangement and stress and conflict should be lessened.

Give lots of advice but be prepared for the fact that it will be ignored. Avoid any sentence beginning, 'When I was your age ...' and if your children do want to talk to you about subjects like sex and drugs, try to be open-minded. Children need to be able to discuss difficult subjects with a parent without feeling embarrassed.

One final word of warning: parents – whether they live together or not – frequently disagree about the way to deal with the children's behaviour or what's happening in or outside the home. If you and your partner want to argue over the children (and who doesn't, occasionally?) make sure you don't do it in front of the children. Always try to present a united front on specific issues that are of concern. Children are experts at picking up any weakness in an argument, and will lose no opportunity to 'divide and conquer'.

Dealing with problems

It is a known fact that relationships do break down, and this can appear all the more devastating when you are in your fifties with your world seemingly collapsing all around you.

Before giving up on a relationship that has been successful for a good number of years, it is worth considering the alternatives very carefully. Resentment can build up over a period of time and even small annoyances can be magnified out of proportion. It is important to think about your life in general, and any other factors that may be upsetting you, as well as perhaps your partner making you unhappy. Now is the time to think about the good points in your relationship rather than just the bad ones. Even though you may consider yourself the innocent party in the breakdown, your own behaviour may also be influencing the situation, especially if there is a third party involved. Infidelity is often a sign of marital unhappiness. The issues need to be discussed and time allowed for healing, if it is at all possible.

Ask yourself a few questions. Are you being reasonable or unfair to your partner? If there are areas of your relationship that are making you unhappy, have you tried to discuss the issues with them? It is important that any issues are 'aired' in a calm manner, without arguing or being aggressive. Imagine life without your partner. Would you really be happier? If things cannot be sorted out between the both of you, it may be worthwhile seeing a professional counsellor, as a third party may be able to put things into perspective for both of you. Going to Relate is a good first step – they will counsel partners in any kind of relationship, married or otherwise, and they are listed in *Yellow Pages*.

Having an affair

Many people can become paranoid about their partner having an affair, especially if they are stressed, depressed or feeling insecure. In fact some people who are constantly voicing their insecurity or accusations may actually cause their partners to seek solace elsewhere, when there was no such problem in the first place.

So how do you know if your partner is being unfaithful? One of the clearest signs that a person has embarked on an affair is a sudden change in habits. They may, for example, bath or shower more often, get a new haircut or start buying new clothes. They may unexpectedly want to lose weight, become fit and start jogging or go to the gym. Some people may suddenly become more romantic at home, presumably in an effort to divert attention away from the affair, or to absolve their guilt. For some, the effect is the complete opposite, as they become callous and indifferent. There may be excuses to be home late more often from work, more frequent nights out with friends, or even trips abroad. They may suddenly enrol in evening classes. Interestingly, they may develop an extra sexual appetite at home – more than they've had for years.

Of course, evidence of any of the above doesn't prove that your partner is having an affair, so don't jump too readily to conclusions. It's just as likely that they may actually have decided to rejuvenate themselves for your sake!

Infidelity means that all is not well in a relationship but the fault is not necessarily all on one side. So if you discover that your partner has been unfaithful and you still want to save the relationship, you will need to be prepared to accept some responsibility for the relationship breaking down. Most people will agree that it is rarely a black and white situation. The important thing is that the problem will not necessarily go away if you ignore it: you have to take some decisive action.

The first thing is to sit down and discuss problems that are bothering you and your partner and find ways to resolve them. Perhaps you may even wish to seek help from Relate or another professional counselling service. If things are not right, then you need to find the element that needs changing – and change it. Try changing yourself too, if you think that will help. Make more effort about your own appearance and attitudes. Take up a new hobby to make yourself more interesting. Relationships can and do recover from one or other partner having an affair and can often be stronger because the circumstances have forced both partners to think seriously about what they have got together – and what they have to lose.

Breaking up

Inevitably some people do split up, and it's usually the choice of one partner rather than both at the same time, making it all the more devastating for the partner who is left behind. Both partners, however, will have to face up to the pain of separation and divorce.

If this should happen to you, it is important at this time to be able to talk through your feelings with a close friend or a family member as this will be a very emotional period. If this isn't possible, then you can talk to your doctor or perhaps find a local support group. You will need to think how your separation or divorce will affect your position among friends and family, especially if you have been a couple for a long time. Facing the world as a single person again is a huge hurdle, and social occasions can be very daunting.

It will be important to overcome any fears, otherwise you can end up becoming isolated, which can turn into a lifetime habit. You should not allow yourself to become trapped in negative emotions such as bitterness, resentment, anger or even feeling sorry for yourself. Although this is easier to advise than do, the sooner you roll up your sleeves and get on with your life the better. This is not the time to sit and brood on your misfortunes: there is a whole new world out there and lots of potential happiness around the corner if you care to go and look for it. Get out of the house every day and meet people. There are plenty of opportunities through work, studying, new hobbies, voluntary work, or sports and leisure activities, so it is up to you to grasp them. It's not always easy but you can do it. Importantly, keep up appearances, even if it's just for yourself.

Be practical about the future. Think all the finances through and get some help from a solicitor, especially if young children are involved, who will still need financial support from the family breadwinner. Ideally choose a solicitor from the Solicitors Family Law Association, whose members are committed to the idea of divorce or separation with as little acrimony as possible. If you have financial difficulties this will add to the burden. Loneliness, tiredness and stress will also tend to make you think about the past and worry about the future. The sooner you can put these pieces together, the sooner you can get on with your life.

Of course, what I've just written in a few paragraphs can take months or years to come to terms with. But the quicker you can move on, the better life will be for you. If you are in your fifties you may start to think that life has passed you by, but that is the exact opposite of the truth. This can be a new beginning and there will be plenty of opportunities to make new friends and to develop new relationships, and choosing a new partner who will be far closer to your needs of today, rather then yesterday.

Leaving one partner and starting afresh with another is never going to be easy. But people do it all the time and usually everyone, including any children involved, will learn to come to terms with the split eventually. But don't expect it to happen quickly – in many cases it may take years.

Give plenty of time for wounds to heal before embarking on any serious relationships, allowing some time (at least a year, the experts say) to establish your sense of identity again. I've already stated that the majority of divorcees get married again and the success rate is far higher the second time around. Perhaps people try a little harder and learn from their previous mistakes – or perhaps they just find someone more compatible.

Of course, the circumstances are completely different if your partner passes away. The grief that follows will be a necessary and traumatic process, and I will cover this area in Chapter 12. But there may be a time when you want to develop a new relationship.

New relationships

Being on your own, especially after many years with the same partner, is not easy for either men or women. Even though you may retain many existing friendships, you may still feel like a gooseberry at parties or social gatherings on your own, simply because other people there are in couples. You may think everyone is looking at you with feelings of sympathy, or pity – or contempt. Of course, this is not the case, but just the way we feel at this time.

It is important to socialise even if you don't really feel like it. Force yourself to go out at least twice a week. Look for hobbies, sports or interests that will take you out of the house and into another environment where you can mix with other people of both sexes. Once you've started socialising on a regular basis you are bound to start meeting potential new partners, although at this time you probably cannot imagine dating again.

After a period of recuperation from your broken relationship you may finally want to seek the company of another person, to regain that feeling of being wanted and sharing one-to-one conversations in a quiet atmosphere, thoughts, ambitions and new experiences. Going out on a date for the first time in many years can be a daunting experience, and it is understandable to worry about what may be expected of you by the other person. Being yourself on a first date isn't the easiest thing in the world to do. You will probably feel insecure about the way you look, what to talk about, or even whether you may be asked to leap straight into bed!

But don't worry. Whether you are male or female, almost certainly you will look a lot better than you actually feel. Confidence is important, so try to be yourself and let your personality shine through. Walk tall, look people in the eye, smile a lot, and you'll make them take notice.

It is important to regard the other person on a first date as a prospective friend rather than a possible partner or new relationship. Be interested, ask questions about their background, hobbies and work, and tell them about yourself. Don't spend time talking about your previous relationship, although you may want to mention any children you have, who will obviously be important to you. Do remember that the other person will probably be feeling as nervous as you are.

Just because you like somebody, don't feel pressurised into having sex. Only consider making love if you know that you are mentally ready for such a commitment. While you may want love, the other person may just want sex, and this is the last thing you will need if you are feeling emotionally fragile.

Be optimistic about your new life. It may seem, at this moment, that you will never find another love. But the pain does pass and bear in mind that if your previous relationship had been right, then you would still be in it. Your new life has every chance of being many times better than the one you've left behind.

Finding the right one

If you think you have met a potential friend who may be a likely partner, beware of embarking on a new relationship too soon, on the rebound. Being alone for a period can be worthwhile and positive, and give you time to shed some of the emotional vulnerability that may be lingering. You don't want to make the wrong choice simply because you don't wish to be alone. Use the time to clarify your attitudes and ambitions.

So how do you know when you've met the right person? Well, your instincts will kick in and you'll probably discover you have a lot in common. You'll have fun, laugh together, respect each other, rely on each other, and have similar goals and values. You'll feel secure and confident of their feelings – and yours.

Everything may seem perfect on the surface, but make sure that you are aware of any lingering relationship your prospective partner may have. Are they still married? Make sure you find out about any possible skeletons in the cupboard, such as gambling or alcohol addiction or money problems. Are your religions compatible? Remember, too, that anyone reaching 50 and starting a new relationship will have 'baggage' that comes as part of the package – work or home commitments, children, family, financial interests. If they have been living alone for some time, they may be set in their ways and find it hard to compromise and adjust to another person – and that may apply equally to you! Be open and honest about your worries, respect the other person's need for their own individuality, and deal with problems in a sensitive but forthright way. Mutual respect and understanding will get you through.

After a period of getting to know the other person, if your instincts say all the right things, then go for happiness and enjoy life while you can. You have many years ahead to do all the new things you want to do – with your new partner.

Sex

As we get older, the old adage, 'A little bit of what you fancy does you good' stands up very well, particularly when it comes to the health benefits of love-making in a close relationship. Bearing in mind that love-making or sexual intercourse can burn a least 100 calories an hour, a moderately active sex life of once a week could burn well over 5,000 calories a year – equivalent to two marathons! – so it provides some very enjoyable exercise. Also research shows that regular sex can actually help to make you look and stay younger.

Apparently it was discovered that couples in a permanent relationship who made love regularly appeared ten years younger than other 'less frequent' couples who were not in a steady relationship.

Other studies show that chemicals released by the brain during sex can act as painkillers, particularly useful for curing a mild headache (!). And an accumulation of feel-good hormones can make sex a great stress-reducing activity, leaving you relaxed, optimistic and smiling.

Then there are the physical benefits. For women, regular sex keeps the vaginal tissue lubricated and strengthens the pelvic floor muscles. For men, regular sex can help to prevent prostate problems in later life. The sexual act literally cleans the prostate gland as semen is squeezed out during orgasm.

Lost libido

Stress and mid-life changes will affect the way we feel about each other, especially if partners are stressed or under pressure at the same time. Boredom, growing apart or sexual difficulties in middle age can seem far worse at this sensitive period and may result in a loss of libido or sexual desire. In turn, a lack of intimacy can occur between couples if sexual activity is off the agenda.

Women going through the menopause will usually experience vaginal dryness that will make intercourse uncomfortable, more difficult and less desirable. Men, because of stress or tiredness after a day's work, may have less desire for sex or may not be able to get an erection. This is quite normal, but a partner may think that this indicates a lack of desire for them personally, and for the wrong reasons. Of course, these problems can be tackled with understanding from either partner. Vaginal dryness can easily be overcome with the use of a lubricant such as K-Y jelly. Another bonus for women after the menopause is that their frequency of orgasm may actually increase and after the menopause many women's sex drive increases, probably due to the fact that both pregnancy and contraception are no longer on the agenda, bringing a new freedom. Men may take longer to be aroused, and may also take longer to reach orgasm, but this can be turned to a love-making advantage for their partner.

Although sexual activity may possibly lessen as we get older, there is nothing to stop us valuing the intimacy of togetherness with a few kisses and cuddles. Provided you and your partner are in good health there is nothing to stop you enjoying sexual intimacy way into old age.

The important key is communication and understanding each other's sexual needs as we get older, with love and intimacy a priority. Always be honest with your partner about your feelings. Discuss any anxieties or problems you may have, which will help to take any pressure off the situation. If you think you have any physical or psychological problems, then don't hesitate to contact your doctor. In most cases the problem can be easily cured.

Impotence

The word means that a man is not able to achieve a hard enough erection to have intercourse. Impotence can sometimes occur in men as they get older for a number of reasons. There can be both psychological or physical causes but all can usually be treated, so it is important to seek help, starting with your doctor.

The most common cause of impotence is anxiety and this becomes a 'Catch 22' situation – anxiety kills all possibility of arousal, and the less you can perform the more the anxiety creeps in. Other psychological factors include problems with a relationship, depression, bereavement, tiredness and stress. But there is also the simple possibility that one partner no longer finds the other attractive. So just because you've been in a relationship for a long time, don't get sloppy with personal appearance and hygeine.

Physiological causes of impotency are more common in older men. These include vascular disorders such as arteriosclerosis (caused by smoking), heart disease and high blood pressure. Diabetes can also often create erection difficulties as can the use of certain drugs, particularly those prescribed for blood pressure, anti-depressants and ulcer treatments. A most common cause that affects all ages is drinking too much alcohol, which may stimulate the desire but has the opposite effect on the performance!

Drugs for treating impotence, such as Viagra, have been developed over recent years. This can be effective in up to 80 per cent of patients. It has to be taken one hour before intended intercourse and will not work unless the man is sexually stimulated. Viagra is a very powerful drug and it is important that it is taken only under the care of your doctor. Possible side-effects include headache, indigestion, dizziness and a flushed face. Other types of medication that work in a similar way to Viagra are available if there are side-effects, and your doctor will have their details.

There are also mechanical aids such as the pubic ring that is placed around the base of the penis, designed for men who cannot sustain an erection for very long. There is also a vacuum pump device, which is placed over the penis and used to create low pressure to encourage an erection.

Depression

Depression is an illness that can affect all aspects of our lives, especially our relationship. When one partner is depressed, the relationship or marriage can become very vulnerable. Anyone who suffers from depression will need all the love, support and closeness they can get from their understanding partner. Depressed people, through no fault of their own, feel withdrawn and have little energy, even to pay any attention to their family or partner. It is easy to wrongly assume that a depressed person no longer loves you or wants to end the relationship.

Depression will affect all the bodily systems and sleep is often disrupted. People who are depressed usually lose all interest in sex, with few exceptions. But sometimes sex or intimacy is the only thing that will give them some comfort and reassurance. With men, tiredness and feelings of hopelessness are common, which may be associated with loss of libido and erection problems. In women, the diminished brain activity that goes with depression tends to be associated with lack of interest in sex. All these problems usually diminish as the depressive illness gets better. Renewed interest in sex may be the first signs of recovery.

Anti-depressant medicines can sometimes interfere with sexual desire. One of the most common side-effects is to make a patient unable to have an orgasm. If this is the case, then ask your doctor for a change in medication.

You can help your partner through this difficult period. Your love and constant support, even when apparently unappreciated, will make a big difference. It is essential that you seek professional help and I have listed some helpful associations at the end of this book. It is important to remember that depression has the same effect as if your partner was recovering from a serious physical illness. They will need time to recuperate and improvement may be slow.

Being around a depressed person can be very draining, so make sure that you also look after yourself in terms of your own pleasure. Your partner may want to stay indoors all the time, despite the fact that it is helpful for them to get plenty of fresh air. If this is the case, get some respite from the situation by going out and socialising, or seeing a film, or having a drink or dinner with a friend. Have a few breaks. Remember that this period of your life will pass, and that your partner will recover. The person that you loved is still there underneath the depression and you are the most important person to help them out of it.

CHAPTER 12

Retirement

If you've only just turned 50, you may not be thinking right now about retirement. But it is something that will come to us all sooner or later, and even if it's not looming on your horizon just yet, it does no harm to start thinking about it and making a few plans. Added to this, many more people are retiring early – through choice or necessity – or being forced to retire, through redundancy. So I make no apology for giving it a full chapter.

Right back at the beginning of this book I mentioned the importance of a positive mental attitude. And whatever the reason for your retirement, if you are going to enjoy it, your attitude will play a crucial part. You can either decide that you have come to the end of your useful life, or you can look forward to starting a new phase, with the time to use all the opportunities it offers. Retirement doesn't have to be the end – it can be a new beginning. But it's up to you.

Make sure your retirement is the beginning of a whole new phase of your life.

Aspiration and ambition are important at any time of life and now is the time to think about further education, new hobbies, travelling or taking up a new sport. Whether you're a single person or one of a couple, you can now enjoy your free time, uninterrupted by children or work. It may take effort to be sociable and involve yourself in activities to make and keep new friends, but you'll be surprised how full your life can be.

Making adjustments

Retirement means change – for the better, we hope, but change nevertheless. It is important to be ready for these changes and to be prepared to adjust to accommodate them.

If you live with someone, you have to adjust to spending more time in each other's company. This may sound like heaven to some, but to others it may be more difficult to handle. Most people like to have a little time and space to themselves every so often, and it can be hard to come to terms with having your partner under your feet day in, day out. Thinking and talking about it together in advance will help a great deal, especially if you make some plans for what you are going to do with the extra time you will have together. Thinking about it on your own will do no harm either – try imagining how you will feel when your partner is driving you mad, hanging round the house all day. You may want to explode with frustration when they start trying to take over what you see as your territory – but it's worth remembering that they may be feeling rather lost and even useless, and desperately in need of something or someone to restore their self-esteem. That could be you. So give it some thought now.

If you live alone, retirement will mean that you have less company and fewer opportunities for social intercourse. If you particularly enjoy a solitary existence, this will not be a problem, but if you are a sociable soul, then you must consider ways of keeping people in your day-to-day life. Again, forward planning is the key – so start looking round before you retire, and don't give loneliness a chance to creep in.

Stay mentally agile

Just because you've given up work doesn't mean you can stop using your brain. Our brains need exercise just as much as our bodies if we are to stay mentally agile. The brain contains billions of nerve cells called neurones, and millions of messages are passed from neurone to neurone every minute of every day, enabling us to convey thoughts and ideas, learn information and retrieve memories. As we age, the neurones stop working as effectively, resulting in some forgetfulness and loss of recall. Experts say that by the time we are in our fifties, some 40 per cent of us will suffer from some age-associated memory impairment.

But, and it is a very important but, studies also show that people who use and exercise their minds on a regular basis not only improve their memory but also their IQ, at whatever age. So there is plenty of hope for us oldies. It is also worth noting there is some evidence that suggests antioxidant foods, which help protect against heart disease, cancer and other illnesses, also protect against illnesses of the brain caused by free radicals (see page 77).

So it's vitally important that you keep mentally active. With so much time suddenly on your hands it can require just as much thought to organise free time in retirement as it did during your working life. Crosswords, brain-teasers, quiz games and regular reading will all help to keep the brain ticking over. And if you want to improve your memory, start to practise and use it every day. You can make this a regular habit, really looking at your surroundings and making mental notes of all the things around you. Use all your senses to see, listen, feel, taste and smell. As an added bonus, you may find that everyday journeys suddenly become a lot more interesting.

Pay attention to minor details. By actively looking and making a conscious effort to take in this kind of information, you start to train your brain to log more details without you even realising. Just like any other muscle, it needs to be exercised regularly.

Keep physically active

Keeping physically active is important – as we get older it can help to stave off physical health problems such as heart disease and osteoporosis, as well as reducing anxiety and stress. Of course, when you finally pack up the working days, you may want to relax and do nothing more than a little gardening, reading a favourite book or playing the odd round of golf, but be aware that your retirement is a new beginning. In general, we are fitter and better off financially than previous generations and, what is more, the opportunities in terms of leisure, activities, hobbies and sport are endless.

Mental exercise

When our children were small, if we were eating out in a restaurant, we would amuse them by taking turns at shutting our eyes while another person asked a question such as 'How many glasses on the table?'; 'What pattern is the tablecloth?'; 'What is in the picture on the wall?'; ' What type of earrings is Mum wearing?' I'm not suggesting that you do the same when out with friends (!), but it is an interesting exercise to close your eyes for a few seconds and see just how much you can remember of your surroundings. It's fun and it will keep your mind working overtime.

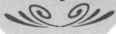

To maintain that fitness why not join the local Ramblers Association and walk in company and make new friends. Also there will be new places to visit or discover. Or if you don't fancy the great outdoors, why not exercise indoors and learn a new dance. Country and Western dancing or line-dancing is a lot of fun and very social (see Chapter 7).

Fill your days

For most of us, our immediate family and friends have always played a major role in how we spend our time. When you are retired or even semi-retired, they will be especially important, as they will give you a sense of belonging and being valued, which you may have taken for granted in a working environment. Make the effort to keep in touch with both friends and family, particularly in the first few months of retirement. Invite them round, get out and visit them and if that's not possible, keep in contact by e-mail, letter or telephone.

If you have children and grandchildren, this is a wonderful opportunity to spend more time with them. You can help your children in practical ways by getting involved with your grandchildren, showing off your parenting skills while giving them a break from their routine, especially at weekends or during holidays. You'll relish your grandchildren's company (and they should enjoy yours) and their parents will appreciate the time to themselves. The big advantage, of course, is that you only have them as long as you want them – and you can hand them back afterwards!

There are some areas of concern to watch out for, however. It will be very tempting, when you suddenly see more of your family, to start trying to tell your children how to bring up their offspring. Do this at your peril. Any comments you do make should be helpful and constructive and offered with the greatest of tact – and preferably only when you are asked for your opinion. Also bear in mind that both your children and grandchildren have their own lives to live, so it may not always be convenient for you to pop round without prior arrangements being made. In the same way, remember that although you now have lots of time on your hands, they may not – so don't expect more from them. And if you're one of the lucky ones who do get more attention, make sure you let them know you appreciate it.

Friendships are important too, so make an effort to stay in touch. Good friendships tend to be less intense because old friends trust each other and can dip in and out of contact as and when it suits. But don't take special friends for granted. Close relationships of any kind need constant nurturing and if you neglect them, you run the risk of their fading away.

Inevitably some friends will move on to pastures new and through a whole gamut of reasons (moving house, divorce, bereavement, etc.) you will end up drifting apart and your circle may be reduced. Consequently it is important that you give yourself the opportunity to make new friends by being involved with new interests and activities that bring you into contact with people. Try to develop younger friendships too, so that they can bring modern concepts into your thinking, helping you to keep touch with the rapid changes in modern life. You will find it easier to move with the times rather than stagnating in old attitudes, and they will benefit too, from the experience and wisdom you have built up over the years.

Have fun

There is little doubt that the more you put into your free time or retirement the more you will get out of it. If you keep your mind and body active you will reap more benefits – you will feel happier and more fulfilled, and will stay healthier and live longer. Not a bad incentive. Some recent research in the UK by a leading insurance company found that most people who have retired in their fifties are now spending their savings on having fun, rather than putting it aside as an inheritance for their children. In fact, it was discovered that three-quarters of the over 50s were treating themselves with holidays, socialising and shopping. Add to this that one in ten of the over 50s now goes out at least three nights a week and you can see that we are not exactly slowing down as we get older!

Retirement does take some planning. It is important to mix activity with relaxation, and home-based activities with outside interests. Follow a leisurely pace and don't burn yourself out. Plan events so that you pursue home interests one day and an outside pursuit the next, so that your pace of life varies from day to day and week to week. Make your days varied, so that you never become bored, and always have something else to look forward to. Keep a diary and make sure that you have entries filled in for the weeks and even months ahead.

Education

It is worth having a look at your local adult education centre for ideas and hobbies. You may fancy learning the language or popular phrases of your favourite holiday destination abroad, where you may now be spending more time. Perhaps you've always fancied trying your hand at some arts and crafts, painting with oils or water colours, even writing that book (there are plenty of creative writing courses). You can also study academic subjects in the comfort of your own home through a correspondence course – there are literally hundreds to choose from and some colleges offer special concessionary prices to mature students.

Your local library will also offer much information as to what's going on in your area and it's well worth making a regular visit to keep up to date with local events, at the same time perhaps using their computer to surf the web! While on the subject of computers, there are some good software programmes that will help you to map out your family tree, which can be quite a rewarding task and will need much detective work. Or if you want some free entertainment, you can always apply for tickets to watch your favourite television or radio shows being made at the studios. Websites for the various television companies will show you how to apply, or you can telephone their helplines.

Catching the IT bug

I personally know several people who had never in their working lives touched a computer (and didn't want to) but, after retiring, were persuaded to invest in one. They've learned how useful it is for internet access, e-mails and writing letters (and operating a keyboard is much easier for anyone who is having trouble writing clearly by hand). All the games on offer (virtual reality golf, grand prix racing, Mastermind, tennis, bridge, chess, etc.) were an added bonus. It's safe to state that in all cases they simply don't know what they would do without their computer now. In fact, as I write, one of these parties is asking for some advice on upgrading or buying a new computer because the one he has is now not powerful or fast enough! You have been warned.

It is never too late to learn something new and, surprisingly, you may think, older people do very well when it comes to learning. This is probably because of the self-motivation and self-discipline that they tend to have, especially when enthusiastic about a brand-new venture. The internet now provides us with a wealth of knowledge around the world and cheap communication through e-mails, so if you have never got to grips with computers now is the time. What a great opportunity! You'll have plenty of time to surf the world-wide web and discover new adventures, both home and abroad, and all at a relatively low price. Special low-price packages include computer, internet access, software, printer and even a scanner to store all your favourite photographs.

Voluntary work

Voluntary work is both popular and rewarding and many retired people feel that they are making a useful contribution to society. Most people find this sort of work far more enjoyable than their former paid employment, usually because there is much less pressure and hours can be organised to fit in around their other activities. Voluntary work can come in many guises. Helping out at a local charity shop or assisting with reading at an education centre or, perhaps, more political pursuits involving local campaigns, wildlife or the environment. Politics can be rewarding too. You could join a national political party so that you can play a role in their campaigning or if you are a little more ambitious and prefer to be more actively involved, think about putting yourself up for election to your local parish or district council.

Financial matters

When you plan your retirement you can work out what the financial situation is likely to be in terms of pension and savings, against everyday outgoings. But for some people, forced early retirement or redundancy comes along without warning and can cancel any forward planning. Then it can become a matter of survival. You can always sell a larger house for something smaller to create a retirement nest egg or to reduce the rent, which is one option (see page 176).

But whatever the reason for your stopping work, it's worth looking at how your spending habits will change. On the positive side, if you are not travelling to and from work, paying for lunches or socialising after work, then there will obviously be some financial saving. On the downside, you may use your car more for travelling to see friends and relatives and your household bills may rise through spending more time at home, especially in the winter months.

If you require some extra income it may be worth considering some part-time activity to help maintain your bank balance. Many people who are made redundant expect to find another job similar to the one they have just left. Nowadays this is unlikely, however, and it may be easier to lower your sights to a part-time job in a completely different field, at least in the short term while you carry on looking for your ideal job, which may possibly take longer than you think. In these circumstances it is best to avoid digging into savings or redundancy payments for as long as you can.

One big holiday

You may now think that life is one big holiday and there's no need to go away, but it will still be important to escape at least once a year to pastures new. Assuming your finances stretch that far, you will now have the opportunity of extending holidays to longer periods, and because you can go at almost any time of year, you can avoid those busy and expensive peak times. This may be the time to visit all those countries you have always wanted to see. You could even have some fun simply planning the details of such trips to be taken at some time in the future. If you have some spare capital, perhaps you could invest in a flexible time-share – the sort that gives you access to holiday venues all around the world. You can take friends or family with you, and the time-share you buy can stay in the family for future generations after you tire of travelling, or you can sell it on at a later date if you need the cash. Beware, though: time-share weeks should not be considered a financial investment.

Of course, you now have the time to explore the countryside around where you live. Many of us never really look at our local area properly. Pretend that you are a tourist visiting the area for the first time. You will probably discover that there are many treats waiting for your visit and all within an hour's drive – castles, museums, gardens, villages, churches, historical architecture and many other areas of interest. Visiting places like this is an economical way of spending a day, especially if you round it off with a stop in some nice little pub or tea shop to give you some much-deserved refreshment.

Whether you choose to travel abroad or at home, the great attraction of retirement is that you can take advantage of out-of-season discounts and accommodation as well as concessionary fares. Many holidays and tours are organised specifically for the over 50s.

Moving house

This may be the time to move, particularly if children have already flown the nest and your house is now too big and expensive to maintain on a day-to-day basis. A smaller home will be easier to look after and cheaper to run. If you own your house, you should be able to realise an extra sum of money to put aside for rainy days, even after paying the removal and solicitors costs. If you are a tenant, a smaller house will still be more economical.

Many people move to be nearer to relatives, or because they want more of a holiday environment, perhaps on the coast or in the country. You may even consider moving abroad and seeking a warmer climate, or consider a bungalow where you will have no stairs to contend with in later years.

It will certainly be important to plan well ahead so that you can be sure any new home will meet all your expectations. The garden will be important if you like pottering around and enjoying the sunshine when it is on offer. Think about the services around you in terms of shops, health care, leisure facilities and public transport. Are they just as convenient as where you live now – or perhaps even better? And don't forget those friends I mentioned, as it may be difficult to make new ones easily. That country or seaside retreat may be wonderful in the summer months but very bleak in the winter. Obtain as much information as possible about the area you wish to settle in. This may be the last time you move house, so you should try to be certain it is the right place for you to live, so that you can look forward to a peaceful and happy retirement, in the long term.

Of course, you may already be thinking about moving to a specially designed retirement village or complex. Each house or flat is built with older people in mind, and there will usually be a warden to look after your needs should you require any help or have to deal with an emergency. Don't be tempted to take this step too early – if you move into a purpose-built retirement home too soon you will probably miss the company of younger people around you, as the inhabitants are likely to be a lot older. But if you are thinking of moving house, it is still worth considering what retirement facilities may be on offer for the longer term in the area where you choose to live (see also Chapter 13 – Elderly Care).

Bereavement – moving on

As we get older and reach middle age, we will more and more frequently experience loss through death of a loved one or close friend. Initially we will lose people who are older than ourselves from our parents' generation, and even our parents themselves. As life moves on, we will be aware of losing people we know from our own generation, certainly when we enter into our sixties and beyond.

It can be helpful in dealing with bereavement if we understand a little about the issues and emotions that it raises. Bereavement can have an important effect on our physical health – indeed, many older people who lose their partner after a life-long relationship will also pass away within a year or so of their partner. Grieving is a normal process and it is important to be able to allow the emotions inside you to have some freedom. Initially it may be difficult to actually accept the loss, and if it is difficult to accept you may feel resentment and anger, or even guilt. People deal with grief in different ways: some simply carry on as if nothing has happened, and others sit alone for hours, feeling that they just cannot move. It is important to confront such emotions and simply talking about the person you have lost can often help to gradually come to terms with your feelings. Be prepared to share your grief with other members of the family and close friends. They'll understand and want to help you.

Many people experience a desire to turn the clock back and be able to talk to their partner, telling them important things that were left unsaid or how much they loved them. This is quite normal and all part of the grieving process. Sharing your thoughts with others can be helpful at this time, telling them what you would have said if you had had the opportunity. Some people visit the grave and 'talk' to the dead person, and some may believe that they see them again.

Moving on without someone you care for can be difficult and create many guilt feelings, which is completely natural. If your relationship was a good one, think about what they would want you to do, and what they would want for you – happiness, surely. So don't feel guilty if you find yourself moving on and enjoying life again. Life must go on and apart from anything you will have a lot of practical things to sort out – sorting out finances, wills, documents, etc., perhaps even moving house. Allow people to help you and don't be afraid to talk, reminisce and express your emotions.

Time really is a great healer, and you will gradually get used to the idea of not having someone close to you any more. It may take a couple of years of adjustment, possibly less. In one way, the feelings of bereavement never end, but they do tend to lighten as the months pass. You will eventually be able to enjoy happier thoughts and memories of your loved one without getting too emotionally upset. People grieve at different rates, so there is no set time-scale for recovery and you may still feel the loss after many years. The important thing is not to let it prevent you from getting on with a normal life again.

It is quite possible that you may require some medication to cope with the initial shock and sleeplessness that bereavement often brings. This should only be considered as a temporary measure because drugs will only delay the natural grief that will eventually come out – and it is probably better to not prolong the agony. Your doctor will help you to deal with any short-term effects. It may take several months to re-establish a normal sleeping pattern and to start getting back to some kind of normality. If it seems to be taking longer, you may be slipping into depression, and you would be well advised to go to have a chat with your doctor. Again, some medication may be helpful as a means of putting life back into perspective. If your doctor suggests this, don't be alarmed – if you broke your leg, you'd expect to have to use crutches. In the same way, mild anti-depressants will help you to cope until you recover your emotional strength.

You may find it helpful to commemorate the person in some way – this can be very comforting, as well as acting as a 'rite of passage' after a bereavement. You could plant a tree in their memory, or buy a painting as a memorial, donate a bench to the local park or golf course, or even give some money to a favourite charity. Doing something lasting in memory of a partner can help you to move on with your life.

You will find that you think a great deal about the person you have lost – but you must also keep thinking about yourself. Keep an eye on your appearance: think about how they would have liked you to look. Give yourself treats, buy a new outfit, have your hair done and, above all, keep going out. It's important to keep up your confidence and to seek opportunities to mix with other people. Although it may seem unthinkable at the time, as the months or years pass, you may even find that you want to consider the possibility of developing a new relationship, especially if you are only in your early fifties or sixties. (See also Chapter 11, Relationships and Sex.)

CHAPTER 13

Elderly Care

I have two reasons for including this chapter: firstly, most people in their fifties will have parents or relatives who may now, suddenly, require help with their day-to-day care. And secondly, because we will all be elderly one day, and as I've already said before, there is great value in forward planning.

In 1995 there were fewer than 9 million people over 65 in the UK – by 2030 there will be about 13 million. And according to recent estimates, the number of people over 60 could rise by 40 per cent in the next 30 years. As someone in their fifties (or older), you are in a position to influence your own longevity and health by adopting lifestyle changes that are covered throughout this book. But it is probably going to be a lot more difficult to influence an 80-year-old after a lifetime of bad habits. So how do we look after our nearest and dearest as they become older – mums, dads, aunts, uncles, even older brothers and sisters?

A sudden decision?

Most of us don't give much thought to caring for an elderly relative, until we are forced to. Then, suddenly, a loved one can no longer manage on their own, or illness strikes and full-time nursing may be required.

According to research by Help the Aged, older people have a very negative view of old age, and fear being isolated and patronised by the young. This presents a real problem: many people are willing to provide unpaid care to elderly relatives, but few elderly people like to receive it. The survey found that older people feel that they are not getting the services they

Caring for elderly parents is something many of us will have to cope with a we get older

179

A familiar story

I can still vividly remember being involved with finding a residential care home for my mother, Rose, when she had just turned 80 years of age. She was quietly determined to remain independent and stay put in her flat, on her own, but she was really not able to look after herself properly on a day-to-day basis. Shopping was a chore, cleaning a burden and cooking something to avoid. She had regular daily help as well as regular visits from family, but once her mobility became difficult, due to bad arthritis, she lost interest in socialising and looking after herself. Having lived on her own for most of her adult life and being fiercely independent, she was totally opposed to the idea of living with her family but she was equally opposed to living in a care home, or 'old people's home' as she put it, which she regarded in the same light as a workhouse from a Charles Dickens novel.

When we finally managed to persuade her to visit several care homes near to where we lived, she was very pleasantly surprised at the facilities and care on offer. Her initial trial stay for a week was, in her words, 'like being on holiday'. The fact that we were now around the corner and could pop in and see her every day was an added bonus. Now she ate regularly, had the company of other residents when she wanted, enjoyed more visits from friends and relatives, and watched most of her favourite TV programmes throughout the day – snooker was her favourite. She even had someone (me) to place that small bet on her favourite jockey or horse on a Saturday afternoon!

need – but most still want to remain independent and live in their own home. They dislike day centres and view residential homes as a last resort. The researchers also reported a widespread feeling of unfairness about the financing of care. Despite agreeing that they should contribute some money towards their own care costs, old people feel it is unjust that those of them who have worked and saved carefully for their retirement will end up using all their own assets to pay for their care, with virtually nothing to show for their years of effort.

Planning ahead

Speaking to friends and colleagues recently, I was amazed at just how many people (especially those of us in our fifties) were facing similar situations. Would Dad cope without Mum if she went first? Could Mum live on her own without Dad? Would they be happy moving in with us if they couldn't cope? Should we be moving to a larger house to cater for the future? There were practical problems to be faced – and the financial side did not bear thinking about. Who's going to pay for what? Who will be responsible for care costs? Will we have to sell Mum's house? Worst of all, we knew that even just asking the questions can lead to distress for all concerned – and always at the most delicate of times.

Planning ahead is, without doubt, the key to elderly care for everyone. It is so much simpler and far less emotional to discuss the 'what ifs' when caring is not yet actually required. All the interested parties, especially the elderly parent or relative, can take part in the decision-making process. After all, it is their future that we will be talking about.

Staying at home

Most elderly people want to remain in their own homes and stay independent, obviously subject to their health and mobility. Though life may become a little more difficult, especially for those living on their own, if the process is gradual, it is quite possible that a few simple modifications around the home could make moving to sheltered or residential accommodation unnecessary in the immediate or foreseeable future. And elderly people tend to cope better in familiar territory than somewhere new and unfamiliar.

An elderly individual who has some self-help difficulties should, in the first instance, speak to their doctor or the local authority social services department. They will arrange for a care assessment to be carried out, to gauge both the degree and form of support that may be required. If a spouse or other family member lives with the person and is able to act as a carer, the carer's needs will also be assessed. But all parties should bear in mind the considerable strain that can be placed on lone carers before making final decisions about staying at home.

Staying at home will be a lot easier with the addition of a few items that will normally be found in a residential or nursing home – from bath seats and grab rails, through wheelchairs and commodes, to telephone amplifiers and stair-lifts. Some of these may be loaned from your local health authority or voluntary organisations such as the WRVS, Age Concern or Help the Aged, so there may not be any great cost involved. There is also an amazing array of cunning gadgets that will help to make basic tasks around the home much easier, as well as hobbies and interests, like reading, needlework or gardening.

You should always get some independent and expert advice before buying expensive and complicated equipment such as stair-lifts or walk-in baths. It is important that the product is designed for the person who is going to be using it, otherwise it may be waste of time and money. Of course, the local authority, subject to financial circumstances (see page 185), may be able to organise

Handy gadgets to look out for

- Kettles fixed to a tip plate for easy pouring
- Different coloured chopping boards to highlight objects being cut
- Plates with inner lips to stop food sliding off
- Colour-coded tap turners for frail hands
- Openers for flip tops, ring pulls and screw-on lids
- Long-handled dustpan and brush
- Electrical sockets fitted at waist height
- Easy-grip electrical plugs
- Electric tipping and lifting chair
- Raised toilet seat
- Bath seats to make sitting and getting out easier
- Hand or grab rails around bathroom or toilet
- Chair with hidden commode
- Portable wheelchair ramps
- Walking frame
- Garden stools on wheels
- Shopping baskets on wheels
- Automatic needle threaders
- Illuminated magnifying glass to help with sewing, etc.
- Large playing cards with holders

home-helps to visit and to do some of the jobs around the house, including cooking, cleaning and shopping.

Many local authorities are able to offer a laundry service and 'meals on wheels' and some provide occasional visitors to give an isolated person some company from time to time.

Personal alarm systems are also available, provided by the local council (for a small charge) or by a private alarm company. These are an excellent idea, even if the elderly person is only left occasionally, for short periods of time. They are very reliable, thanks to modern technology, and there is no need to be technically minded to operate them – you just press a button and the alarm is raised at a central switchboard. Some even have a phone-back facility so that you can explain what the problem is. A mobile telephone is also a worthwhile purchase. With falling call charges and pay-as-you-go tariffs, keeping in touch has never been easier.

Choosing a care home

There may come a time when your elderly relative has to leave home because they can no longer cope on their own. This is the really tricky bit. Think back to when you last went house-hunting. You knew when you'd found the one you wanted – it just felt right. The same feeling applies when seeking a room or apartment in a sheltered accommodation, residential care or a nursing home. A word of warning: remember who you are choosing for. You may be putting in all the legwork, shopping around, but even if you think you've found the ideal place, your elderly relative may not share your enthusiasm. If possible, you should take them with you to look at the available places. This home is for them, not you, and their criteria may be completely different from yours.

Bear in mind that if your relative qualifies for a fully-funded nursing home (see page 185), he or she may not have a choice of which home to go into. They will also have their state pensions and benefits reduced, as they would if they were staying in an NHS hospital.

The first priority will be to decide which type of care home meets their needs. Note that a dedicated residential home cannot cope with nursing, and a nursing home will not provide residential care, unless it is dual-registered. So the term 'care home' can be a little ambiguous – and unhelpful.

Sheltered accommodation, for example, ranges from accommodation specially designed for older people (featuring mobility aids, personal alarms and a resident warden) to more complex establishments that cater for the very frail, requiring high levels of support, more comparable with a residential home. Residential homes offer the kind of back-up provided by a competent, caring relative at home – providing meals, administering medicines and helping with washing, bathing, dressing and visits to the loo. Many homes help with incontinence, while some are registered and equipped to deal with the physically disabled, as well as the mentally impaired.

Nursing homes provide a much greater level of care. They have the facilities and expertise to look after those suffering from severe confusion and immobility, as well as many other needs.

For good measure, there are dual-registered care homes which will cater for both residential and nursing care. These are usually larger establishments and are ideal for those people who do not require nursing at the moment but may do so at a later date, as the disruption of moving homes at a critical time of their life will be avoided. They are also the perfect solution for a couple who both require care, but at different levels. Here they can receive both types of care at the same time, still being together.

Remember that the care home you choose need not be in the area where the elderly person lives. Local authorities have reciprocal arrangements with others around the country, so that residents may change areas to be nearer relatives. A list of care homes in your area may be obtained from your doctor or an organisation such as Age Concern or Help the Aged.

The next step is to look at the establishments themselves and to see if they will have any vacancies at a time to suit future decisions.

First impressions are important. Look for a happy, pleasant atmosphere and a homely smell. If, on the other hand, you are conscious of strong, lingering aromas possibly redolent of a public convenience, then go no further than the front door – carry on to the next care home on your list.

In making your choice, much comes down to common sense. For instance, if a large number of residents seem to be confused whereas the person you are checking the home for is particularly alert, the chances are that the home will be unsuitable. You should look for residents who are of similar abilities and age groups to your relative.

Note how the staff behave towards the residents. Do they stop and chat? Do they genuinely care, or do they give the impression that they are too busy to stay any longer than they have to? Many care homes are on very tight budgets and will certainly not be over-staffed. Are there any male staff in evidence? Women residents usually outnumber the men, but most like to see a male face around to give some balance. Mealtime arrangements are important too. There should be at least two main menu choices at both lunch and dinner, plus a standby, such as an omelette and salad, should other offerings be unacceptable to some. Menus should be rotated on a monthly basis, or more often.

You must inspect all of the living accommodation. Look at all the reception rooms and then ask to see the residents' private rooms. They should be sufficiently roomy to spend time in and entertain, as well as accommodate any private furniture. Are educational and social activities held on a regular basis? Will a pet be welcome? Are there special events like Christmas parties and lunches, and do residents have a cake on their birthday?

Many care homes print their covenant in their brochures and also hang it on the wall for all to see but it is better to make an appointment to see someone in charge and ask them a few questions. Check that they are happy to invite residents to take part in any decisions affecting their care and daily living arrangements. They should allow visitors to call at any time and be prepared to offer meals for a small extra charge. Some may also offer overnight accommodation. Make sure they can provide special diets and requests where appropriate. Ask what their procedure is for complaints – they should be promptly investigated and satisfactorily resolved without fear of reprisal.

Of course, you will probably be assured that all of this is available, but for it to work in practice depends a great deal on willing employees who know what they are doing. Find out what the turnover in staff has been in the last couple of years (ask one or two of the residents – they will tell you). The fewer the changes, the happier the team will usually be.

Once you've made a short list, go back for a second visit – or a third – to ensure your impression remains favourable. And, if possible, arrange for the would-be resident to stay for a trial week or weekend. Many homes offer temporary respite care to give full-time home carers a break, so this can make an ideal opportunity for you to see how things work out.

Who pays for what?

At the moment, many potential elderly care residents are means-tested to see if they qualify for financial help with their care. Note, however, that all nursing and medical care costs are covered by the NHS.

In the UK, people with assets worth less than £19,000 will qualify to have their care home costs paid by the local authority. Personal care and accommodation must be paid by those with assets above the £19,000 limit. People who will pay their own care fees need not involve the local authority at all. But if it is likely that their funding will run out or they may need assistance at some time in the future, it is still advisable to get an assessment. If the local authority is going to contribute towards the costs, they should tell you the amount that they will pay and give you details of the care homes in your area within their price range. If you are unable to find a home to meet your relative's needs (this is not the same as meeting their wishes!) within their price limit, they are obliged to increase their limit to do so.

As stated previously, you can arrange to move out of your area into another local authority's area, although their existing council will still be responsible for the costs. This arrangement applies to England, Wales and Scotland but excludes Northern Ireland. Bear in mind that in Scotland all care is free. This can be a problem when moving from a low-cost area to a more expensive area as a reciprocal arrangement may be more difficult. But a local authority is obliged to pay the extra if an assessment recommends that the person be moved, perhaps to be close to family, or because of cultural or religious needs.

If your relative has less than £19,000 but more than £11,750, then this asset will be converted into an assumed weekly income, referred to as a tariff income. Any assets below £11,750 will be ignored. A spouse's savings or income will not be taken into account for asset purposes, but the authority can approach the spouse and ask that they make a contribution. No other relative or family member can be asked to contribute.

If your relative has more than £19,000's worth of assets, they will be expected to refund the full cost of their care fees. If they own their own home, its value will be counted as capital, as will shares, savings, etc., which can sometimes be a blow if they were hoping that their children would inherit the property. But there are some important exceptions to this rule that are well worth knowing (see panel).

Your property as an asset

- The property as an asset should be disregarded when calculating the cost of the first 12 weeks of permanent care.

- If a husband, wife or unmarried partner continues to live in the house, then its value will not be counted in a capital assessment.

- If a relative aged 60 or over continues to live in the house, then its value will not be assessed.

- If a relative under 60 who is incapacitated lives there, the value will not assessed. Also if the resident has responsibility for a child under 16 and the house is their main home, it will be not be counted.

- A local council may also ignore the value of a house if a carer lives there – although this is at their discretion.

- If the person going into a care home is classed as a temporary resident (i.e. they are expected to stay less than 52 weeks), then the local authority should ignore the house as an asset.

- If the home is co-owned with another person, the council may also take this into consideration.

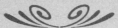

Be aware that it is illegal to make over a property or any savings to another person in order to qualify for financial help from a local authority. This is called deprivation of assets. If a council believed that this has been done deliberately they have the power to presume that the assets belong to the original owner.

The local authority will take a person's savings and income into account when working out any payment towards a care home's fees. On the plus side, they must also make an allowance for personal expenses. This is set by the government each year.

If you have any problems trying to identify your particular situation it would be sensible to take advice. Organisations such as Help the Aged and Age Concern have a wealth of experience in these matters and would be a good first port of call (see Old age, page 205).

Covering the cost

With the prospect of paying out considerable sums, you may want to consider some kind of forward financial planning. Some insurance policies are specifically designed to help protect capital and enable money to be left for the rest of the family, and the earlier they are taken out, the less they cost. In many cases, a house, which is probably the largest asset, can provide an annuity policy, which may be purchased by using all or part of the house value. This will enable a person to stay in their home as long as they wish. It can also provide a regular income (for both individuals if a couple is involved) and will still allow people to move house and take the annuity with them.

I would recommend that you get personalised financial advice, preferably from an independent source. Organisations like the excellent Nursing Home Fees Agency will provide expert advice according to the circumstances. (See page 205.)

A final word

Whether your relative stays at home or is in residential care, you should try to make sure that every effort is taken to ensure that they remain as healthy as possible. One particularly important aspect of this care is nutrition.

In old age optimum nutrition is vital. Eating moderately is desirable and a varied and well-balanced diet is essential. Most care homes realise this and their menus have been devised and balanced to provide the maximum vitamins and minerals within a varied diet. We have covered a healthy diet already in detail (see Chapter 4), but it is worthwhile defining some of the areas that need special attention for the elderly – especially when living at home.

During the ageing process several changes take place. For example, energy requirements decline as physical activity decreases, but the need for vitamins and minerals becomes more essential. The body's metabolism slows down and the lean body mass (muscle tissue) is reduced. Although less protein may be needed, less efficient digestion and assimilation means that the same amount of protein is required in the diet. Loss of appetite is common – this may be due to a number of causes, such as apathy (especially if living alone), poor teeth, a dry mouth and a reduced sense of taste and smell (exacerbated by zinc deficiency). A lack of taste and smell may also lead to unhealthy dietary changes as the sufferer tends to move towards stronger tasting and less healthy foods like crisps (chips), snacks, salted foods and sweets. As a result, even with a reduced appetite, the elderly can still put on more weight, increasing the risk of degenerative diseases such as cardiovascular disease and diabetes.

As the elderly tend to have smaller appetites they can easily miss meals without noticing. It is important to encourage them to eat little and often – four or five small meals a day may be better rather than three full-sized meals. Vitamins, minerals and fibre are important, so encourage them to eat plenty of fresh fruit and vegetables each day, including fruit juice. Bear this in mind if you are doing the shopping for them, adding treats that they may not necessarily buy for themselves. Encourage them to eat wholemeal bread, rice and pasta, and to include pulses in their meals. Foods rich in essential fats should be regular fare. Oily fish, such as mackerel, herring, sardines and salmon, are ideal sources of these, as well as protein, and are also light and digestible.

Thirst also decreases with age, but it is still important to drink plenty of water every day, to help encourage the removal of waste from the body and to prevent dry skin. Dehydration is common among the elderly due to the inability to recognise the need for fluid. The situation is made worse by the increasing use of diuretics, being afraid to drink to avoid frequent visits to the toilet, and even physical difficulties such as hands that tremble and are too weak to turn on taps. Make sure that your relative has a source of fresh water ready to hand at all times. If they don't enjoy plain water, try introducing them to a variety of herbal teas to make the taste more interesting.

Make sure they have plenty of company too – the elderly try a little harder when eating with their friends and family. Check that they can chew well – poorly-fitting dentures or bad teeth may be making this difficult. Make the meals interesting, varied and colourful, to encourage them to copy when cooking for themselves. And if you feel that your elderly relatives are not eating as well as they should, persuade them to take a multivitamin and mineral supplement every day.

As well as diet, keep an eye on their mobility. Encourage them to remain both physically and mentally active to retain all their faculties as long as possible. Gentle exercise such as walking, dancing and bowls will be of major benefit and many elderly people enjoy swimming – local leisure centres usually provide special sessions for them. It is never too late to try and improve our health.

CHAPTER 14

Rapid Results

Nowadays everyone wants the quick fix, the instant response. I've spent most of this book explaining that improving your health and prolonging your active life is not quite that simple, but this chapter offers you the nearest thing to a short-cut version. If you follow this simple advice – 50 ways to being fab at 50! – in a matter of just 50 days, you could be on the road to a new you.

1 Think about diet, fitness and lifestyle

You'd be hard put to find a medical professional who doesn't agree that the combination of healthy diet, exercise and lifestyle play a vital role in reducing the effects of ageing, and the prevention of many diseases. Consequently you will add more years to your life, and more life to your years, by adopting simple measures or philosophies to help reduce the effects of ageing.

2 Take a positive attitude

How old do you feel? Do you feel any different from the way you felt five or ten years ago? Our psychological age is our own perception of how old we think we are. If you continue to be active and continue to do things you have enjoyed for many years, you are more likely to feel and stay younger. A positive attitude can dramatically improve both your physical and emotional well-being. People who are happy are not only more pleasant to be with, they are less likely to suffer from stress-related disorders and high blood pressure. Laughing also actually helps to boost the body's immune system. Be happy and positive; smile and laugh: it really is good for you.

Here are some routes to quick results to encourage you towards that longer healthier life.

3 Take regular exercise

Everybody, including me, talks about fitness and how good it is for you. The thing is to put aside at least 30 minutes a day for some form of exercise. The more you do it regularly, the more you will want to do it. So start with something that's easy and comfortable. Walking is, without doubt, nature's natural exercise and if you can manage 30 minutes day (15 minutes there and back), this could change your life. The most important message is to do something every day so that it becomes a habit – and you can do it wherever you are. Walk instead of using the car or public transport; use the stairs regularly instead of lifts and escalators.

4 Remove stress from your life

People who suffer from stress will be more susceptible to illness and accelerated ageing – this is a fact. So recognising stress and anxiety, and dealing with it, will be an important part of improving your life and longevity. Stress can be a hidden enemy; it may not be the stress itself that causes damage, but the inability to cope with it. Not being able to cope with stress can lead to anxiety and depression. Now is the time to look at your life and remove all the negatives. Make a concerted effort to remove the causes of any stress, for the sake of your long-term health and well-being.

5 Stand up straight

We can look ten years younger by a change of posture. The older we become, the more rounded and smaller we can appear, so simply holding ourselves tall and upright will take years off – and you will feel the difference. Your clothes will hang better and you will even appear slimmer. A good posture is also good for your health, as a correct stance, coupled with exercise, will help to increase bone density and protect the spine as you become older. Hold your shoulders back and lift your head high, as if someone is pulling the crown of your head upwards on a string. Your tummy will immediately appear flatter.

6 Keep up with fashion

Don't try to look too young – and don't let your look age you. As we get older, we can easily get caught in a comfortable time-warp with both clothes and hairstyles – wearing similar outfits and haircuts that we have worn for the last 20 years. So with fashion and style in mind you should buy clothes that suit your figure, with emphasis on the good parts and less emphasis on the bad.

7 Get a new hairstyle

A smart hairstyle makes you look and feel better, so experiment. Try a new cut and a new colour, if you like. Get some professional advice and remember when making your colour choices that as you grow older, both your skin and hair lose some colour, so you may need to go lighter, not darker to cover up the grey.

8 Feed your skin on the inside ...

Despite the advertising claims of many skin products, it is unlikely that any product will halt or reverse the signs of ageing skin. What we put inside our bodies is probably more important than the products we use on the outside. Both water and nutrients are vital for the repair and growth of skin, and ensuring they are part of your regular diet will help to give and retain a smooth and youthful complexion.

9 ... and protect the outside

It is never too late to start protecting your skin from the sun, so reach for the sunblock. Smoking will also accelerate the appearance of wrinkles – so give up if you can. Use moisture-rich products for your particular skin type and protect your skin from harsh weather. Simply steaming your face over a bowl of hot water with a towel around your head will cleanse it and help to plump up the skin with moisture and unclog pores.

10 Look after your eyes ...

Your eyes are the first thing people notice about you, so take good care of them. A soothing eye mask is a nice way of resting red, tired eyes, or there is nothing more soothing than a couple of cold cucumber slices laid on closed eyelids. When you need to soothe dry eyes use lubricating eye drops. If you wear glasses, update the frames to suit the shape of your face, hair colour and complexion. Modern frames can take years off the way you look.

11 ... and your teeth

There is no quick way round brushing and flossing your teeth every day to keep them in top condition and free of plaque. If they are stained, visit a hygienist for advice on cleaning, and if they are crooked, see an orthodontist. Modern techniques and applications can work wonders with alignment and colouring.

12 Try Botox instead of brunch

Cosmetic surgery is a quick – if drastic – method of physically removing signs of ageing. A recent development, used for the removal of lines and wrinkles, is Botox treatment. It takes as little as ten minutes to perform, which is why it is called the lunch-hour treatment. A tiny amount of purified botulism bacteria (Botox) is injected into a specific area near the crease or wrinkle and binds on to the nerve, causing a temporary paralysis of the corresponding muscle, which has the effect of removing or lightening any creases in the skin. It's expensive, though, and will only last a matter of months.

13 Cut back those years

A more serious cosmetic surgical procedure for a younger look is a face-lift. Under general anaesthetic the skin is cut from behind the hairline down to the front of the ear, then around the fold behind the ear and over to the back of the head. Fat and double-chins can be removed and the jawline firmed up. You can get astonishing results in a matter of weeks, but if you overdo it you'll look ridiculous. It's expensive, too.

14 Act as old as you feel

A rather less drastic way to start looking and feeling younger is to check how you perceive yourself. Ageism can sometimes start with our own thinking. If you start to think of yourself as older, you subconsciously see yourself as others want to see you, which may be little to do with how you feel in terms of physical and mental fitness. Suddenly you may feel older than you actually are, and this may be reflected in your demeanour and body language. Be positive and reflect how you feel about yourself, rather than what may be expected of you by others.

15 Keep your brain in trim

Learning is a great way of keeping the mind in trim – and can be lots of fun. How about learning a language or popular phrases for your favourite holiday destination? Perhaps some arts and crafts, painting with oils or water colours, even writing that novel. You can also study a more academic course in the comfort of your own home through a correspondence course, with hundreds to choose from. Of course, the world-wide web provides as much information as you can absorb, subject to your desire. And if you don't have a computer now's the time to buy a package and get on-line.

16 Relieve stress – try sex

Research shows that regular sex can actually help to make you look, feel and stay younger, because couples in a permanent relationship who make love regularly appear physically younger than 'less frequent' couples. Sex is also a great stress-reducing activity – leaving you relaxed, optimistic and smiling. Then there are the physical benefits, apart from the obvious exercise. For women, regular sex keeps the vaginal tissue lubricated and strengthens the pelvic muscles. For men, regular sex can help to prevent prostate problems in later life. The message is clear – keep at it.

17 Less sex? Try more love!

Sexual incompatibilities may become an issue for the first time in our middle years, with boredom, tiredness or routine fading a relationship. Partners may be worried about their attractiveness or there may be physical problems. Women may become dissatisfied and men feel threatened. But all is not doom and gloom. Most couples survive difficult patches and end up closer than before. Love-making, although less frequent, may become more loving, enjoyable and carefree. Make an effort to be more loving – and who knows where it may lead.

18 Balance your food intake

Making a few subtle changes to your diet can help to strengthen your resistance to many illnesses, from the common cold to heart disease and some cancers. Make sure you eat the right balance of protein, carbohydrates, fibre, fats and minerals. The average person eats only half the recommended amount of fruit and vegetables, but almost double the recommended intake of fat. Bear in mind that we do not put on weight because we eat too much, but because we eat badly.

19 Stop cheating on your diet

The best way to stop yourself cheating is to keep a food diary. It will give you an overview of your eating and drinking habits, and will help you analyse areas that you may need to change for the sake of your health or to maintain your correct weight. To start you off, try keeping a note of everything that you eat or drink over a seven-day period.

20 Get plenty of vitamins

Vitamins are vital organic compounds that we need for bodily growth, function, repair and maintenance. There are two groups of vitamin – water-soluble and fat-soluble. Water-soluble vitamins include the B complex group and vitamin C, and they need to be replenished daily. Fat-soluble vitamins, which include A, D, E and K, are stored in the body for longer periods. Women especially are thought to need extra nutrition at various stages of their lives, while slimmers and vegetarians may not be getting enough nutrients. Start eating a balanced diet with plenty of protein, fresh fruit, vegetables and cereals to make sure your body gets all the vitamins it needs for good health.

21 Minerals are a must

A diet containing a balanced variety of foods (meat, fish, dairy products, nuts, cereals, vegetables and fruit) will not only supply vital vitamins, but will also provide all the minerals that we need, which are essential for our health and well-being. Minerals comprise approximately six per cent of our body weight and form the greater proportion of our bones and teeth. A poor nutritional status, in particular with relation to protein, zinc, iron and vitamin levels, can lead to an inefficient immune system. If you think you're not getting enough, take a good supplement.

22 Drink water

Water is the elixir of life – our essential ingredient. Water plays an important role in our diet, well-being and longevity. Our bodies consist of two-thirds water and it assists the body's cooling system, aids digestion, removes toxins, helps to keep our joints mobile and supple, and will improve the texture of the skin. Water will also help decrease your appetite if you want to lose a little weight. An adult should drink at least six to eight glasses of water a day, depending on weight, age and level of activity. Ideally use filtered or bottled water, or tap water in a filter jug. Get into the water habit and drink throughout the day.

23 Tipple for pleasure – not thirst

An alcoholic drink now and then is thought to be good for you, but in moderation. The official recommended maximum we should drink is 28 units (men) or 21 units (women). A unit is 8 grams (10 ml) – a glass of wine, half a pint of beer or a single spirit. To help cut down it is a good idea to drink only when eating, then the drink is metabolised at a slower rate, combining with the food to produce fewer fat reserves. Another tip to cut alcohol intake is to drink every other day. Drink water to quench your thirst and then sip your tipple for taste and pleasure.

24 Cut the caffeine

Although small amounts of caffeine have been linked to alertness and brain activity, large amounts are associated with high blood pressure. Caffeine is also addictive. So it will be worthwhile cutting out or down on its intake. The first step is to drink only decaffeinated tea and coffee. Avoid colas and fizzy drinks. If you usually drink tea and coffee all day, substitute with water and introduce other hot drinks such as herbal tea.

25 Know your cholesterol

Achieve 'good' cholesterol by avoiding food containing saturated fats and eating plenty of fish, pulses, fruits, vegetables, and even a regular glass of red wine. Olive oil is a 'good' fat and ideally should be used for salad dressings and cooking. Bad cholesterol comes from saturated fats in meat (remove fat and skin), some cooking oils, butter, lard (shortening), cream, etc. Learn to recognise which foods to avoid and adjust your diet accordingly.

26 Throw away the salt

Too much salt is bad for us, especially as we grow older, being associated with high blood pressure (hypertension). Replace salt with healthier flavour-enhancers like lemon, Tabasco, peppercorns or fresh herbs. If you can't eat food without a dash of salt, then add a small pinch at the cooking stage rather than at the table, or use low-sodium alternatives. Avoid take-away foods – they contain more than their fair share of salt, sugar and fat. Remember, you could cut out salt completely and still receive your share of sodium naturally through other foods – and you'd be much healthier.

27 Get your head round labels

Understanding a food label is important, so that you can pick and choose what you are adding to your diet. All food labels have to contain certain elements of statutory information. These are the manufacturer's name and address, a list of ingredients in descending order of weight, and 'use by' or 'best before' dates. Most manufactures give the basic information on how much energy, protein, carbohydrate and fat a food contains per 100 g and, sometimes, per portion. Some labels also give information on saturates, sugars, fibre, sodium, vitamins, minerals, etc. When shopping, check all the labels.

28 Eat fruit and vegetables

Antioxidants help prevent oxygen reacting with molecules in our body in ways that could cause damage, possibly encouraging some cancers and heart disease. The damage is caused by 'free radicals'. Our environment, including pollution and smoking, can help to create excessive amounts. We can help protect ourselves against free radicals when we eat antioxidant nutrients in the form of vitamins A (beta-carotene), C and E, as well as the mineral selenium. Most fruit and vegetables are likely to have been treated with chemicals so clean thoroughly or remove skin. Eat organic whenever you can.

29 Build up your immunity

Many factors can undermine our immune system. Modern forms of food processing, chemical residues in food and the over-use of antibiotics are just some of the reasons contributing to our immunity inefficiency. Our modern environment, with its central heating, air conditioning and atmospheric pollution, can influence our susceptibility to viral illnesses. Eating a healthy diet, taking regular exercise and getting a regular good night's sleep help to boost and maintain our immune system.

As stress can also weaken our immune system, it is important that we reduce stress levels not only through exercise, but by taking time out to relax.

30 Breathe properly

Breathing correctly can help us to reduce stress levels, boost immunity, and even help with depression or sleepless nights. We tend not to breathe deeply enough, which leads to a poor exchange of oxygen. When we breathe we should use our diaphragm, which lies at the bottom of the chest cavity. Use this muscle to breathe in and out without allowing your upper chest to rise and fall. Aim to breathe slowly, smoothly and deliberately, achieving about ten or 12 deep breaths a minute.

Do this at least once a day to get into the habit of breathing correctly, especially when outside in the park or countryside, and enjoy the difference.

31 Make fish a favourite

Essential fatty acids (EFAs) should form an important part of a healthy diet to help prevent diseases, especially of the cardiovascular system. Essential fatty acids cannot be manufactured by the body, so it is essential that we obtain the right amount from our food. Oily fish (especially sardines, mackerel, herring, trout, salmon, tuna, pilchards, kippers and sprats) and flax and pumpkin seeds are highly concentrated sources of omega-3 essential fatty acids, which are polyunsaturated oils closely linked to immunity efficiency, and should be included in the diet once a week. Omega-3 EFAs make the blood less likely to clot, reducing the risk of a heart attack or stroke.

32 Relax to reduce the strain

Stress, apart from adversely affecting our immune system, depletes our levels of vitamin C, which are needed to help detoxify the body of harmful substances. Relaxation and meditation with deep breathing exercises, as well as therapies such as aromatherapy and reflexology, are also excellent stress-relieving aids. Cut down drinks that act as stimulants, such as coffee, tea and cola drinks, replacing them with calming herbal teas such as camomile, blackberry, lemon balm and peppermint.

33 Get a good night's sleep

Undisturbed sleep encourages efficient cell repair and renewal, rejuvenating and revitalising both the body and mind. Bad sleepers are usually more stressed, have less energy and are more likely to suffer from high blood pressure and high blood cholesterol. Stimulants, such as coffee, tea, cola, chocolate, nicotine, spicy food and alcohol, should be avoided as much as possible, especially late in the evening. Milky bedtime drinks will calm the mind and encourage sleep and regular exercise during the day will also encourage healthy sleep patterns. Lavender is a well-known aid to relaxing, so try a few drops of lavender oil on your pillow, or a sachet of lavender under it. Make sure that your bed is comfortable and that the room is well ventilated.

34 Walk more

Studies show that we walk far less than we should, especially as we get older. Due to the increase of gadgetry in our lives we work less and less. We use cars, taxis, trains and buses more and more. Also escalators, lifts, electric doors, remote controls, television and internet shopping, home deliveries . . . the list is endless. Walking is probably the most ideal low-impact, low-risk and low-cost activity. It is well documented that walking can have massive health benefits. Even walking at a moderate pace for as little as 30 minutes a day can significantly improve your cardiovascular system. Your heart will become stronger, your lungs more efficient and blood pressure can normalise.

35 Work out with a video

It is easy to exercise regularly in your own home, so you have no excuses about being too cold or wet outside. Exercise equipment, keep-fit videos and even magazines and books offer programmes for all abilities in the comfort of your bedroom or lounge. Videos are an excellent start as you can buy exercise regimes to suit various age groups and fitness levels, and they supply easy-to-follow instructions, with music to work to. Don't worry if it all seems too complicated at first: after watching a video a few times you will quickly learn the routine and be able to run through without thinking, just using the music.

36 Go for a swim

Water sports are a gentle way of introducing your body to more exercise – the water supports your weight and there is therefore less stress on the joints and muscles. Swimming uses most of the main muscle groups, so is one of the best sports for a gentle all-round fitness. It suits all age groups and provides a workout that will help improve the condition of your heart and lungs. If you find swimming a bit boring, you can try aqua-aerobics – exercise classes in the pool. Aqua-aerobics is a great way to get fit without having to feel too energetic. As you would expect, movements are slow, but because the water is resistant, you actually work harder than you realise.

37 Come dancing

Why not enjoy a regular turn around the dance floor to keep fit? Even if your footwork isn't all that fancy, your local dance school should soon have you stepping in the right direction. Singles, couples and groups are all welcome and there is a variety of dance styles to suit everyone, such as ballroom, tap, modern, Latin American, line-dancing and rock 'n' roll. Each dance can be a fun form of exercise and very sociable at any age.

38 Stretch for safety

There are some fitness regimes that require less effort, utilising various movements, stretches and co-ordination. These are particularly useful for someone with restrictive movement, and can be beneficial for older people who may be less mobile. Three of the better known stretch and exercise regimes are yoga, Pilates and t'ai chi. Yoga, through various postures, helps to strengthen muscles, improve flexibility and well-being. Pilates teaches breathing, body mechanics, balance, co-ordination, strength and flexibility. T'ai chi uses a series of slow movements, which can actually build up stamina and strength, especially when practised daily.

39 Book a bit of luxury

If you want to kick-start your health fitness regime with a little pampering, you could give yourself an incentive and a treat at the same time by booking a break at a health farm. Before you make your choice decide what your main priorities are: pampering and relaxing; sports and fitness; pools and saunas; healthy eating; or natural and complementary therapies. A three-night stay midweek will be cheaper than a weekend and many health farms now offer one-day visits, with prices depending on what you choose to do. Sharing a room with a friend is also a cheaper option than going it alone.

40 Watch your weight

Is your waist measurement a little more than it was ten years ago? We know that weight gain tends to occur with increasing age, particularly between the ages of 30 and 45. Women tend to increase their body weight until their mid-sixties. Obesity is now the major cause of many of the diseases that try to see us into an early grave – arthritis, depression, high blood pressure, cancer, diabetes, heart disease, hiatus hernia, osteoarthritis, kidney disease and strokes. Several studies confirm that health and good nutrition co-exist – when one deteriorates so does the other! Get into the habit of weighing yourself regularly – and do something about those extra pounds.

41 Check your BMI

So how much should you weigh? Most doctors use the BMI (Body Mass Index) to measure whether you are considered overweight or not. To calculate your BMI, you divide your weight in kilograms by your height in metres squared. Being classed as overweight is defined as having a BMI of more than 25. Over 30 and you are clinically obese. Nearer 35 would be registered as severe obesity and you should have a chat with your doctor. Recent thinking considers waist sizes for simplicity of diagnosis, and female patients with waist sizes over 35 in (86 cm), and over 40 in (100 cm) for men, are considered to be at risk. Check your size now – and if it's more than it should be, take immediate appropriate action.

42 Start a long-term diet

If you think you're overweight, don't reach for the latest fad diet or slimming pills. This is one area where you should avoid short-term solutions. Healthy balanced eating, with a few simple changes in your lifestyle, can work wonders without the need of any special diets. We take in calories when we eat and burn calories through our energy. If we can manage to eat a little less of fat and sugar, or burn a few more calories than normal, then you will lose weight. So perhaps a few minor eating adjustments (minimise snacking) and a little more physical activity (more walking) could do the trick. Men should eat no more than around 1,500–1,700 calories a day, and women should eat a maximum of 1,200–1,300.

43 Book a health check

People over the age of 50 should have a check-up at least once a year, especially if a particular complaint needs to be kept under observation. Regular screening and check-ups will also give you peace of mind. Some people can even stress themselves into an early grave by worrying about illnesses that they do not actually have! So the message is to be safe and sure, remembering that when it comes to illness, the old adage that prevention will always be better than cure stands the test of time. The average health screen will take about an hour and could easily save your life.

44 Read up about the menopause

The menopause occurs at an average age of around 50 years – the range is actually 47 to 52 years of age. There are many views of how women should deal with the menopause and it is an important time of their life. The menopause is a natural event and shouldn't be treated as an illness. It can be easy for a doctor to prescribe extra hormones (HRT) and for a woman to make the best of it. But this may be the appropriate time for women to prepare for the menopause before it occurs, with diet and lifestyle playing an important role in how the menopause will actually affect them.

Many women advocate the natural way of dealing with the menopause and if you follow this route, the sooner you start the better.

45 Consider hormone replacement therapy

So should you take HRT? It certainly works for hot flushes, night sweats and vaginal dryness. It reduces the incidence of broken hips and it helps with dry skin and hair. There are some disadvantages with HRT, with minor side-effects occurring in around 15 per cent of users. These include breast tenderness, weight gain, nausea, headaches, itchy skin, rashes, mood swings and fluid retention. Go and talk to your doctor about it – if you're one of the women who are suited to HRT, you'll feel a difference in a lot less than 50 days. If you prefer a natural approach, see Chapter 8.

46 Check yourself out – women

Most women who experience breast problems tend to make a link with cancer, but in fact nine out of 10 cases are usually benign (non-cancerous). Most experts agree that the best way to minimise the risk is to become familiar with your breasts. Examine them carefully every month and always report any unusual changes to your GP. Although it is common to have minor lumps or bumps in your breasts, particularly just before menstruation, in the majority of cases, they are due to benign breast changes, which can make the breasts feel generally lumpy.

47 Check yourself out – men

Just as women need to check their breasts for lumps, men should also get to know their testicles a little better. They should get used to looking for any lumps and bumps, tenderness or enlargement, preferably while having a bath or shower when the body is warm, soapy and relaxed. Each testicle should be gently rolled between thumb and forefinger to feel for any lumps or swellings. Contact the doctor if any differences are noticed.

48 Natural therapies

If you've got a niggling minor ailment but you don't want to go to the doctor, consider a natural therapy instead. There are many types of natural therapies available to suit many ills and ailments, especially for over 50s. When selecting a therapy, check the qualification of the practitioner. Have a preliminary chat with the therapist, explaining why you think you may need the treatment and to see if he or she has any experience in treating a similar condition with other patients. Always keep your doctor informed of your actions.

49 Make time for yourself

We all need time for ourselves and very few of us bother to make it. If you have a busy routine you need a break now and then, but even if you're retired, you may find that you fill your whole day with a complete timetable of tasks, duties and chores. It's important that you allow yourself some time for pleasure too – it has great value for your long-term health. At least an hour a day is ideal, but an hour a week is better than no time at all. Think about how much you pay a tradesman for an hour's work. Get into the habit of finding time for yourself, even if you spend it reading in the bath.

50 Stop smoking

New Year, a birthday or an anniversary is a good time to quit smoking as it provides an incentive to stretch that success as long as possible. But any time will do – today is fine. The first week will probably be the worst, but you can offer yourself all sorts of special rewards as you progress, especially with the money you'll be saving. There are many aids to help you kick the habit, but joining up with a friend will help, providing support for each other. You will have cleared all the nicotine from your body in a couple of days, and you'll notice an improvement in your senses of taste and smell within weeks. And in just six months your lungs will have increased their capacity by up to 10 per cent.

Further Reading

Atkins, Dr Robert, *Dr Atkins' New Diet Revolution* (Vermilion)

Marsden, Kathryn, *The Complete Book of Food Combining* (Piatkus Books)

Montignac, Michael, *Dine Out and Lose Weight* (Montignac Publishing)

D'Adamo, Peter, *Eat Right 4 Your Type* (Century Books)

Eyton, Audrey, *The Complete F-Plan Diet* (Penguin)

Podell, Richard, *The G-Index Diet* (Warner Books)

Katahn, Martyn, *The Rotation Diet* (Bantam Books)

Sears, Barry, *The Zone Diet* (HarperCollins)

Humphries, Carolyn, *The Hugely Better Calorie Counter: Essentials* (W. Foulsham & Co. Ltd) 0-572-02745-0

Humphries, Carolyn, *The Hugely Better Slimming Plan: Essentials* (W. Foulsham & Co. Ltd) 0-572-02842-3

Humphries, Carolyn, *The 7-Day Hay Diet Plan* (W. Foulsham & Co. Ltd) 0-572-02406-1

Zebroff, Karen, *A Gentle Introduction to Yoga* (W. Foulsham & Co. Ltd) 0-572-02802-4

Kyriazis, Dr Marios, *The Look Young Bible* (W. Foulsham & Co. Ltd) 0-572-02729-X

Further Information

Please note that inclusion in this list does not constitute a recommendation.

Cosmetic surgery

British Association of Aesthetic Plastic Surgeons
35–43 Lincoln's Inn Fields
London WC2A 3PE
Tel: 020 7405 2234
www.baaps.org.uk

British Association of Cosmetic Surgeons
17 Harley Street
London WIN 1DA
Tel: 020 7323 5728

Harley Medical Group
6 Harley Street
London W1G 9PD
Tel: 0800 917 9000
www.harleymedical.co.uk

Lanark Centre
10 Harley Street
London W1G 9PF
Tel: 0800 028 7093

Transform Medical Group
22a Wimpole Street
London W1M 8LD
Tel: 0500 595959
www.transform-medical.co.uk

Diet and nutrition

British Nutrition Foundation
High Holborn House
52–54 High Holborn
London WC1V 6RQ
Tel: 020 7404 6504
www.nutrition.org.uk

SlimSeekers
PO Box 66
Tunbridge Wells TN4 9WZ
Tel: 01892 535300
www.slimseekers.co.uk

World Health Organisation
www.who.int

Exercise and fitness

Body Control Pilates Association
6 Langley Street
London WC2H 9JA
Tel: 020 7379 3734
www.bodycontrol.co.uk

British Council for Chinese Martial Arts
110 Frensham Drive
Stockingford
Nuneaton
Warwickshire CV10 9QL
Tel: 0906 302 1036
www.bccma.org.uk

British Heart Foundation
14 Fitzharding Street
London W1H 6DH
Tel: 020 7935 0185
www.bhf.org.uk

British Wheel of Yoga
25 Jermyn Street
Sleaford
Lincolnshire NG34 7RU
Tel: 01529 306851
www.bwy.org.uk

Health Farm Directory
Spas Research Fellowship
Tower House
Tower Road
Tadworth
Surrey KT20 5QY
www.thespasdirectory.com

Ramblers Association
2nd Floor
Camelford House
87-90 Albert Embankment
London SE1 7TW
Tel: 020 7339 8500
www.ramblers.org.uk

Your body's health

Arthritis Research Campaign
Copeman House
St Mary's Court
St Mary's Gate
Chesterfield
Derbyshire S41 7TD
Tel: 0870 850 5000
www.arc.org.uk

Breast Cancer Care
Kiln House
210 New Kings Road
London SW6 4NZ
Tel: 020 7384 2984
www.breastcancercare.org.uk

BUPA Wellness
Battle Bridge House
300 Gray's Inn Road
London WC1X 8DU
Tel: 0800 616029
www.bupa.co.uk

Cancer BACUP
3 Bath Place, Rivington Street
London EC2A 3JR
Tel: 0808 800 1234 (office)
www.cancerbacup.org.uk

Diabetes UK
10 Parkway
London NW1 7AA
Tel: 020 7424 1000
www.diabetes.org.uk

Menopause Help
www.menopausefacts.co.uk

**National Medical Examination Network
(Medxscreen)**
Poolgate House
68 Park Street
Lincoln LN1 1UR
Tel: 01522 878878
www.nationalmedical.co.uk

National Osteoporosis Society
Camerton
Bath BA2 0PJ
Tel: 0845 450 0230
www.nos.org.uk

Prostate Cancer Charity
3 Angel Walk
Hammersmith
London W6 9HX
Tel: 0845 300 8383
www.prostate-cancer.org.uk

Smoking – Giving Up
Tel: 0800 1690169
www.givingupsmoking.co.uk

Smoking Quitline
Tel: 0800 002 200

Stop Smoking Clinic
www.medicdirect.co.uk/clinics

Stroke Association
Stroke House
240 City Road
London EC1V 2PR
Tel: 0845 303 3100
www.stroke.org.uk

Natural therapies

Academy of Systematic Kinesiology
16 Iris Road
West Ewell
Epsom
Surrey KT19 9NH
Tel: 020 8391 5988
www.kinesiology.co.uk

Bach Flower Remedies Centre
Mount Vernon
Bakers Lane
Sotwell
Oxon OX10 0PZ
Tel: 01491 834678
www.bachcentre.com

British Acupuncture Council
63 Jeddo Road
London W12 9HQ
Tel: 020 8735 0400
www.acupuncture.org.uk

British Chiropractic Association
Blagrave House
17 Blagrave Street
Reading
Berkshire RG1 1QB
Tel: 0118 950 5950
www.chiropractic-uk.co.uk

British Homeopathy Association
15 Clerkenwell Close
London EC1R 0AA
Tel: 020 7566 7800
www.trusthomeopathy.org

British Hypnotherapy Association
67 Upper Berkeley Street
London W1H 7QX
Tel: 020 7723 4443

British Massage Therapy Council
17 Rymers Lane
Oxon OX4 3JU
Tel: 01865 774123
www.bmtc.co.uk

British Medical Acupuncture Society
12 Marbury House
Higher Whitley
Warrington
Cheshire WA4 4QW
Tel: 01925 730727
www.medical-acupuncture.co.uk

British Osteopathic Association
Langham House West
Luton, Bedfordshire LU1 2NA
Tel: 01582 488455
www.osteopathy.org

British Reflexology Association
Monks Orchard, Whitbourne
Worcester WR6 5RB
Tel: 01886 821207
www.britreflex.co.uk

Colonic Association
16 Drummond Ride
Tring
Hertfordshire HP23 5DE
Tel: 01442 827687
www.colonic-association.com

Craniosacral Therapy Association
Monomark House
27 Old Gloucester Street
London WC1N 3XX
Tel: 07000 784735
www.craniosacral.co.uk

Feng Shui Society
377 Edgware Road
London W2 1BT
Tel: 07050 289200
www.fengshuisociety.org.uk

General Council and Register of Naturopaths
Goswell House
2 Goswell Road
Street
Somerset BA16 0JG
Tel: 08707 456984
www.naturopathy.org.uk

General Osteopathic Council
Osteopathy House
176 Tower Bridge Road
London SE1 3LU
Tel: 020 7357 6655
www.osteopathy.org.uk

Guild of Naturopathic Iridologists International
94 Grosvenor Road
London SW1V 3LF
Tel: 020 7821 0255
www.gni-international.org

Hydrotherapy Association
1 Wanborough Business Centre
West Flexford Lane, Wanborough
Guildford, Surrey GU3 2JS
Tel: 01483 813181

Institute for Optimum Nutrition
13 Blades Court
Deodar Road
Putney
London SW15 2NU
Tel: 020 8877 9993
www.ion.ac.uk

International Federation of Aromatherapists
182 Chiswick High Road
London W4 1PP
Tel: 020 8742 2605
www.int-fed-aromatherapy.co.uk

Maharishi Ayurveda Health Centre
24 Linhope Street
London NW1 6HT
Tel: 020 7724 6267

National Institute of Medical Herbalists
56 Longbrook Street
Exeter
Devon EX4 6AH
Tel: 01392 426022
www.nimh.org.uk

Register of Chinese Herbal Medicine
Office 5
Ferndale Business Centre
1 Exeter Street
Norwich NR2 4QB
Tel: 01603 623994
www.rchm.co.uk

Shiatsu Society UK
Eastlands Court
St Peters Road, Rugby
Warwickshire CV21 3QP
Tel: 0845 130 4560
www.shiatsu.org

Society of Teachers of the Alexander Technique
1st Floor, Linton House
39–51 Highgate Road
London NW5 1RS
Tel: 020 7284 3338
www.stat.org.uk

UK Council for Psychotherapy
167–169 Great Portland Street
London W1W 5PF
Tel: 020 7436 3002
www.psychotherapy.org.uk

Personal relationships
General Register Office
Office for National Statistics
Cardiff Road
Newport NP10 8XG
Tel: 0845 601 3034
www.statistics.gov.uk

Relate
Herbert Gray College
Little Church Street
Rugby, Warwickshire CV21 3AP
Tel: 0845 456 1310
www.relate.org.uk

Solicitors Family Law Association
PO Box 302
Orpington
Kent BR6 8QX
Tel: 01689 850227
www.sfla.co.uk

Old age
Age Concern
Astral House
1268 London Road
London SW16 4ER
Tel: 0800 009966
www.ace.org.uk

Centre for Policy on Ageing
19–23 Ironmonger Row
London EC1V 3QP
Tel: 020 7553 6500
www.cpa.org.uk

Help the Aged
207–221 Pentonville Road
London N1 9UZ
Tel: 020 7278 1114
www.helptheaged.org.uk

Nursing Home Fees Agency
St Leonard's House
Mill Street
Eynsham
Oxford OX29 4JX
Tel: 01865 783000
www.nhfa.co.uk

Women's Royal Voluntary Service
WRVS Head Office
Milton Hill House
Milton Hill
Steventon
Abingdon
Oxfordshire OX13 6AD
Tel: 01235 442900
www.wrvs.org.uk

Index